Fertility Decline in Developing Countries, 1960–1997

Recent Titles in
Bibliographies and Indexes in Geography

A Bibliography of Geographic Thought
Catherine L. Brown and James O. Wheeler, compilers

Climatic Effects on Individual, Social, and Economic Behavior
Philip M. Parker

Fertility Decline in Developing Countries, 1960–1997

An Annotated Bibliography

Compiled by
Samuel Agyei-Mensah

Bibliographies and Indexes in Geography, Number 3

GREENWOOD PRESS
Westport, Connecticut • London

Library of Congress Cataloging-in-Publication Data

Agyei-Mensah, Samuel, 1961–
Fertility decline in developing countries, 1960–1997 : an annotated bibliography / compiled by Samuel Agyei-Mensah.
p. cm.—(Bibliographies and indexes in geography, ISSN 1044–8349 ; no. 3)
Includes bibliographical references and index.
ISBN 0–313–30242–1 (alk. paper)
1. Fertility, Human—Developing countries—Bibliography.
I. Title. II. Series.
Z7164.D3A34 1999
[HB1108]
016.3046'32—dc21 98–51612

British Library Cataloguing in Publication Data is available.

Library of Congress Catalog Card Number: 98–51612
ISBN: 0–313–30242–1
ISSN: 1044–8349

First published in 1999

Greenwood Press, 88 Post Road West, Westport, CT 06881
An imprint of Greenwood Publishing Group, Inc.

Printed in the United States of America

The paper used in this book complies with the Permanent Paper Standard issued by the National Information Standards Organization (Z39.48–1984).

10 9 8 7 6 5 4 3 2 1

Contents

Preface vii
Acknowledgements ix
Journal Sources xi
Abbreviations xiii

1. Concepts and Theories of Fertility Decline 1

2. Fertility Decline in Latin America 13

3. Fertility Decline in Asia 35

4. Fertility Decline in Sub-Saharan Africa 73

5. Fertility Decline in Developing Countries: General Literature 115

Author Index 127
Subject Index 135

Preface

The study of fertility decline has witnessed a profound growth over the last three decades. This growth is evidenced by the voluminous amount of literature that has emerged on fertility decline during this period. Despite the breadth of literature on the subject, our knowledge of the decline is scattered in numerous publications making references difficult to come by.

This was the problem I faced during the initial stages of my doctoral dissertation in 1994, as I began looking for literature on fertility decline in the developing world. I realised that there was no published bibliography of fertility decline in the developing countries that covered the three major regions: Latin America, Asia and Sub-Saharan Africa. In addition, published bibliographies on fertility in developing countries, particularly those on Sub-Saharan Africa, have focused on issues such as explanations for high fertility in the region, or general issues pertaining to reproductive health and family planning issues.

With the emergence of fertility declines in the greater part of the developing world, a bibliography is needed that enhances our knowledge of the emerging fertility trends. The objective of this book is to provide an annotated bibliography that will encompass fertility declines in the developing world. The bibliography adopts a regional perspective and examines fertility declines in three geographical regions of the world: Latin America, Asia and Sub-Saharan Africa, covering the periods 1960 to 1997. The bibliography also provides readers with an introductory background on concepts and theories underlying fertility declines. Even though the study seeks to be as comprehensive as possible, I do not claim that it is exhaustive as I have had to select documents for inclusion in the work.

The bibliography is unique in several respects. The material is derived from extensive sources including student dissertations, books, and research papers. The bibliograhy also makes extensive use of references from leading population journals such as *Population and Development Review, Demography, Population Stud-*

ies, and Studies in Family Planning. The broad geographical scope of the study makes it beneficial to students and researchers in the developing world, while the three decades covered make it useful in assessing temporal changes. Indeed, the bibliography will be an invaluable asset for population experts and students interested in carrying out research on fertility decline in the developing world.

In each chapter, the citations are arranged alphabetically by the last name of the first author. Author and subject indexes are provided at the end of the bibliography. The bibliography is organised into five chapters. Chapter one gives a review of some of the concepts and theories underlying fertility decline. It is intended to guide the reader in understanding the major theories and concepts underlying fertility decline. Chapter two looks at fertility declines in Latin America. In chapter three, attention is focused on fertility declines in Asia. In chapter four we look at the declines in Sub-Saharan Africa, while chapter five looks at general literature on fertility declines in developing countries.

Acknowledgements

A number of institutions and individuals have been helpful in the course of this book. The following libraries have been the major sources of literature: the library facilities at Christian Michelsen Institute, Bergen, Norway, the Rockefeller and Science Libraries of Brown University, U.S.A., the Library Services of the Norwegian University of Science and Technology (NTNU), and the Library of the Regional Institute for Population Studies, University of Ghana.

The following individuals have been helpful in the course of the work. Prof. Asbjorn Aase of the Department of Geography (NTNU) and Cynthia Harris, my editor, who responded so quickly and enthusiastically to the book.

Journal Sources

Acta Sociologica
Africa
African Journal of Reproductive Health
African Population Paper
African Review
African Studies Review
African Study Monographs
Agricultural Economics
Ambio
American Economist
Annals of the Association of American Geographers
Applied Geography
Artha Vijnana
Asia Pacific Economic Review
Asia Pacific and Policy Review
Asia Pacific Population Research Reports
Asian Economic Journal
Asian Journal of Economic and Social Studies
Asian Pacific Economic Literature
Asian and Pacific Population Forum

Boletin Demografico
Botswana Notes and Records
Bulletin of the Ghana Geographical Association

China Journal of Population Science
China Population Today

Demography

Economic Development and Cultural Change
Economic Geography
Economic and Political Weekly
Economist
Environment and Conservation
Environmental Impact Assessment Review
Estudios Demografiscos y Urbanos
Eugenics Quarterly

Family Perspective
Forum for Applied Research and Public Policy
Forum for Development Studies

Genus
Geoforum
Geografiska Annaler
Geographical medica
Geographical Review
Geography

Habitat International

Health Policy and Planning
Health and Population Perspective and Issues
Health Transition Review
Human Organization

International Family Planning Perspective
International Journal of Health Services
International Journal of Sociology of the Family
International Migration Review
International Sociology

Journal of Biosocial Science
Journal of Comparative Family Studies
Journal of Development Economics
Journal of Family History
Journal of International Development
Journal of Marriage and the Family
Journal of Social Development in Africa
Journal of South East Asian Studies
Journal of University of Science and Technology

Kieler-Geographische-Schriften
Korea Journal of Population and Development

Middle East Journal
Milbank Memorial Fund Quarterly

New York Times
Nordisk Samhallgeografisk Tidsskrift
Norsk Geografisk Tidsskrift
Notas de Poblacion

Outlook on Agriculture

Pakistan Development Review
Population (Paris)
Population Bulletin
Population and Development Review
Population and Environment
Population Impact Project Newsletter
Population Index
Population Research Leads
Population Research and Policy
Population Studies
Population Today

Reproductive Health Matters
Revista Geografica
Rural Sociology

Science
Scientific American
Social Biology
Social Forces
Social Science and Medicine
Social Science Research
Sociological Forum
Sociological Inquiry
Sociological Perspectives
Statistics in Medicine
Studies in Family Planning
Svensk geografisk arsbok

World Development
World Health Forum
World Health Statistics Quarterly

Zeitschrift fur Bevolkerungswissenschaft

Abbreviations

AIDS	Acquired Immune Deficiency Syndrome
CACM	Central American Common Market
CPS	Contraceptive Prevalence Survey
DHS	Demographic and Health Survey
GDHS	Ghana Demographic and Health Survey
GFS	Ghana Fertility Survey
GSS	Ghana Statistical Service
HIV	Human Immunodeficiency Virus
IRD	Institute of Resource Development
IUSSP	International Union for the Scientific Study of Population
KCPS	Kenyan Contraceptive Prevalence Survey
KDHS	Kenyan Demographic and Health Survey
NPC	National Population Council
PIP	Population Impact Project, University of Ghana
PRB	Population Reference Bureau
PSTC	Population Studies and Training Center Brown University
RIPS	Regional Institute for Population Studies University of Ghana
TFR	Total Fertility Rate
UN	United Nations
UNICEF	United Nations Children's Fund
WHO	World Health Organisation
WFS	World Fertility Survey

1

Concepts and Theories of Fertility Decline

001. Becker, G. S. (1960). An economic analysis of fertility. In *Demographic and Economic Change in Developed Countries*, Universities-National Bureau Conference Series, no. 11, pp. 209-31. Princeton: Princeton University Press.

The author introduces the New Home Economic model of fertility. The model states that under modern conditions, the net costs of having a child are positive, therefore people would have a child only if they thought that doing so would result in the child being valued for its own sake.

002. Becker, G. S. (1981). *A Treatise on the Family.* Cambridge: Harvard University Press.

The study introduces the Chicago Columbia model of fertility decline. The model, like most economic models, assumes that preferences are fixed and endogenous; thus, it explains fertility differences over time and across individuals and groups in terms of a single explanatory category, differences in opportunities.

003. Blake, J. (1985). The fertility transition: Continuity or discontinuity with the past? In *IUSSP International Population Conference, Florence 1985*, Vol. 4, pp 393-405 Liege: IUSSP.

This paper explores the concept of fertility transition, and questions the theoretical basis of the distinction between natural and controlled fertility.

004. Bongaarts, J. (1978). A framework for analysing the proximate determinants of fertility. *Population and Development Review*, 4, 1, pp. 105-132.

The study came up with four principal proximate determinants of fertility: the proportion of women married or in sexual unions, contraceptive use and effectiveness, the prevalence of induced abortion, and postpartum infecundability.

005. Bongaarts, J. & S. Watkins (1996). Social Interactions and Contemporary Fertility Transitions. *Population and Development Review*, 22, (4), pp. 639-682.

This article provides a special kind of diffusion study based on the movement of fertility ideas through social networks that are either natural or specifically created for that purpose.

006. Boserup, E. (1985). Economic and Demographic Interrelationships in Sub-Saharan Africa. *Population and Development Review*, 113, pp. 383-398.

The author introduces a crisis led transition hypothesis that links economic crisis to fertility change.

007. Cain, M. (1983). Fertility as an Adjustment to Risk. *Population And Development Review* 9. No 4, pp. 688-701.

This article provides a framework for understanding fertility change that places importance on security concerns of parents and the value of children as insurance against risk, and for viewing such concerns as an important influence on the reproductive behaviour of parents in developing countries.

008. Caldwell, J.C. (1980). Mass education as a determinant of the timing of fertility decline. *Population and Development Review*, 6, No 2, pp. 225-255.

The author argues that mass education is critical in inducing the onset of fertility transition. He introduces a number of mechanisms by which education could affect fertility, three of which are demand related. The three demand related mechanisms are the reduction of the child's potential as a worker, increased schooling costs, and the fact that schooling makes the child more dependent.

009. Caldwell, J.C. (1982). *Theory of Fertility Decline.* New York: Academic Press.

This book develops a wealth flows theory of fertility decline based on the idea that the decline in fertility comes from the emotional nucleation of the family, a change that may come by either economic or cultural forces.

010. Caldwell, J.C. (1997). The Global Fertility Transition: The Need for a Unifying Theory. *Population and Development Review*, 23 (4), pp. 803-812.

The author stresses the need for a unifying theory of fertility decline in order to enhance our understanding of fertility transitions.

011. Carter, A. T. (1995). Agency and fertility. For an ethnography of practice. In Susan Greenhalgh (ed.). *Situating Fertility. Anthropology and demographic inquiry,* pp.55-85. Cambridge University Press.

The study has two main objectives: First, to show that the concepts of agency that have been employed in theories of fertility change do not work. Second, an alternative view of agency is proposed to free us from the sterile opposition between passive and active decision-making.

012. Carlson, G. (1966). The decline of fertility: innovation or adjustment. *Population Studies*, Vol. 20, No 2, pp. 149-174.

The author classifies explanations of fertility decline into one of two categories: innovation diffusion or adaptation. Carlson argues that the fertility transition is best conceptualised as an adjustment process in which birth control is employed by couples to adjust their fertility to a new set of structural and motivational forces.

013. Casterline, J.B., R.D. Lee & K.A. Foote (eds.). (1996). Fertility in the United States. New Patterns, New Theories. *Population and Development Review*, Supplement to Vol. 22, 337 pages.

This book consists of a collection of articles on fertility in the United States. The collections are meant to stimulate and refresh our thinking on fertility theories, trends and patterns in the United States. They provide new perspectives on theories of fertility that are not only of relevance to the United States but also to other third world settings.

014. Cleland, J. & C.Wilson. (1987). Demand Theories of the Fertility Transition: An Iconoclastic View. *Population Studies*, 41, pp. 5-30.

The study based on the World Fertility Survey conducted in the developing world in the 1970s finds little support that structural changes affecting family economy are responsible for bringing or initiating fertility decline. Instead they argue that the declines are more consistent with ideational factors.

015. Coale, A. (1973). *The demographic transition: International Population Conference* Vol. 1, pp. 53-73. International Union for the Scientific Study of Population, Liege.

The study provides three conditions as necessary for the onset of fertility transitions.

First, fertility must be within the calculus of conscious choice. Second, reduced fertility must be advantageous, and third, effective techniques of fertility reduction must be available.

016. Cochraine, S.H. (1979). Fertility and Education. What Do We Really Know? *World Bank Staff Occasional Papers* no. 26. Baltimore: The John Hopkins University Press.

The author explores the relationship between education and fertility. Cochraine argues that we could expect either a positive or negative relationship depending on a country's level of development and on whether one is dealing with the education of men or women and with short-run or long run effects. She suggests that the strongest and most consistent effect of education is the knowledge and attitudes it fosters toward the use of contraception.

017. Demeny, P. (1992). Policies Seeking a Reduction of High Fertility: A Case for the Demand Side. *Population and Development Review* 18, pp. 321-332.

A distinction is made between the demand and supply arguments for fertility reduction. The author argues that the dichotomy that separates these two fertility reduction policies are unnecessary since one policy influences the other.

018. Donaldson, L. (1991). *Fertility transition: The Social Dynamics of Population Change.* Blackwell. 227 pages.

This book provides a theory of fertility decline based on the idea that changing cultural norms affecting family life-styles and use of time affects fertility decline.

019. Dyson, T. & M. Murphy. (1985). The Onset of Fertility Transition. *Population and Development Review.* Vol. 11, pp. 399-440.

Based on examples drawn mainly from the developing world, the author advances the thesis that the onset of fertility transition is often preceded by fertility increase.

020. Easterlin, R. (1966). On the relation of economic factors to recent and projected fertility changes. *Demography,* 3, pp. 131-153.

The study introduces the relative income hypothesis of fertility decline which states that the standard of living one experiences during childhood is the base from which one's chances as an adult are evaluated, or in other words, the decision to have a child will be influenced by material aspirations nurtured during adolescence.

021. Easterlin, R., R. Pollak, M.L. Watcher. (1980). Toward a more general

economic model of fertility preferences. In R.A. Easterlin (Ed.) *Population and Economic Change in Developing Countries.* Chicago University Press pp. 81-135.

The author introduces the Pennsylvania model of fertility change. The model postulates that consumption experiences in childhood and adolescence determine an individual's later consumption standards, and hence the values that help govern fertility decisions.

022. Egero, B. (1994). Reproductive change is as a social process. In B. Egero & M. Hammaskjold (eds.), *Understanding reproductive change: Kenya, Tamil Nadu, Punjab, Costa Rica,* pp 9-30. Lund University Press, Lund Sweden.

The author reviews papers presented in the volume on reproductive change in Kenya, Tamil Nadu, Punjab, and Costa Rica. The focus of the study is not only to assess reproductive change per se. More importantly, it addresses reproductive change as a social process influenced by both internal and external factors.

023. Freedman, R. (1979). Theories of Fertility Decline: A Re-appraisal. *Social Forces* 58, 1, pp. 1-17.

The study examines the classic demographic transition theory and its applicability in the West as well as in some developing countries. Based on these experiences, the author shows that the transition to low fertility can also occur in situations not envisaged in the classic demographic transition theory.

024. Goldscheider, F. (1995). Interpolating Demography with Families and Household. *Demography,* 32, No 3, pp. 471-480.

The author stresses the importance of the individual, family and community level influences on fertility behaviour.

025. Greenhalgh, S. (1990). Toward a political economy of fertility change: Anthropological contributions. *Population and Development Review.* Vol. 16 no 1, pp. 85-106.

The essay highlights the contributions of cultural anthropology to fertility change, stressing conceptual factors that have been overlooked in the enthusiasm for anthropological methods. It provides a preliminary formulation of the basic precepts of a political economy of fertility and enumerates some of the obstacles that must be overcome before a genuinely interdisciplinary approach to demographic political economy can take root and flower.

026. Greenhalgh, S. (ed.). (1995). *Situating Fertility. Anthropology and*

Demographic Inquiry. Cambridge University Press. 304 pages.

In this book, ten anthropologists and two historians develop new cultural and political approaches to human reproduction. They draw on new ethnographic and historical research and informed by contemporary anthropological theory. The book elaborates a culture and political economy of fertility that incorporates the place of culture and history, gender and power in reproductive life.

027. Greenhalgh, S. (1995). Anthropology theorises reproduction: Integrating practice, political economic, and feminist perspectives. In Susan Greenhalgh (ed.) *Situating Fertility. Anthropology and Demographic Inquiry*, pp. 3-28. Cambridge University Press.

The author places demographic theories of fertility decline into five main groups: classic transition theory, the post-classic fertility transition theories, institutional approaches, contemporary fertility transition theories, political economy, feminism, and practice approaches.

028. Henry, L. (1961). Some data on natural fertility. *Eugenics Quarterly* 8, pp. 81-91.

The author provides one of the early meanings of the natural fertility concept. He uses the word natural fertility to distinguish between couples living in stable sexual unions who do not deliberately engage in behaviour to limit the number of their births in response to a target or desired family size.

029. Kaplan, H. (1994). Evolutionary and wealth flow theories of fertility: Empirical tests and new models. *Population and Development Review* 20, no. 4 pp. 753-791.

The study tests the empirical validity of Caldwell's wealth flows theory in three traditional settings in South America. No support for Caldwell's theory was found. A new theory of fertility decisions based upon evolutionary ecology is posed focusing on trade-offs between fertility and the reproductive value of offspring, and between care of, and resource investment in children.

030. Kates, R.W. (1995). Presidential Address. Labnotes from the Jeremiah Experiment: Hope for a Sustainable Transition. *Annals of the Association of American Geographers,* 85 (4), pp. 623-640.

The study examines among other things the demographic transition, and argues that development, family planning efforts, and culture all contribute to the decline, with development playing the major role.

031. Kertzer, D.I. (1995). Political-economic and cultural explanations of demographic behaviour. In Susan Greenhalgh (ed.). *Situating Fertility. Anthropology and Demographic Inquiry*, pp. 29-52. Cambridge University Press.

The author stresses the importance of a political economy approach to fertility decline and links this to empirical studies from Europe and Africa.

032. Kirk, D. (1996). The Demographic Transition. *Population Studies*, 50, 3 pp. 361-387.

This article provides a theoretical basis for understanding fertility change. It traces the transition from its pre-modern regime of high fertility and high mortality to a post-modern regime of low fertility and low mortality. It concludes that the transition is a universal phenomenon in which every country can be placed within a continuum.

033. Kreager P. (1991). Early modern population theory: a reassessment. *Population and Development Review* 9, No 3, pp. 411-435.

The author finds the current discussion on western demographic transition as a wider part of ideational theory puzzling, considering the fact that the main tenets of ideational theory were once shared by early modern writers such as Hobbes, Machiaveli, Bodin, Locke, Rousseau and Starkey. According to Kreager, the fact that a less prominent role was given to reproduction in this calculus than is given today, should not disguise the extent to which the period established a way of thinking about the causes of population change and its role in development that remains the core of modern approaches. In effect Kreager sees ideational change as an old label that has been revived to reflect present day contemporary events.

034. Landers, J. (1992). Historical Epidemiology and The Health Transition. Introduction: *Health Transition Review* Supplement to Volume 2, pp. 1-27.

The study offers one of the most recent critiques of the demographic transition theory looking at examples from the West as well as some developing countries. The importance of political and cultural factors in influencing fertility changes in developing countries are highlighted.

035. Lesthaeghe, R. J. & J. Surkyn. (1988). Cultural dynamics and economic theories of fertility change. *Population and Development Review* 14, No 1, pp. 1-45.

The study provides a theoretical basis of the ideational component of fertility change with empirical examples from Europe. The study argues that the two most salient features of the Western ideational change have been the processes of secularisation and individuation.

036. Malmberg, B. (1994). Malthus and beyond. An essay based on a seminar series held at the Swedish Royal Academy of Science. *Nordisk Samhållgeografisk Tidsskrift*, no. 19, Sept, pp. 75-82.

The author argues that a transition to low fertility levels in developing countries would entail a radical restructuring of women's social and economic conditions.

037. Mason, K. O. (1986). The Status of women: Conceptual and methodological issues in demographic studies. *Sociological Forum* 1, No. 2 pp. 284-300.

The author proposes a set of hypotheses concerning female status and fertility. In Mason's view, women's education and their position in the family and household are among the most important determinants of fertility. These factors affect women's autonomy, economic independence and social status, which in turn influence child supply, child demand and child costs.

038. Mason, K. O. (1992). Culture and fertility transition. Thoughts on theories of fertility decline. *Genus*, 48, No. 3-4, pp. 1-13.

The article attempts to clarify current thinking about the determinants of fertility transitions. It draws readers attention to the ambiguities surrounding the usage of the terms culture, ideational and diffusion.

039. Mason, K.O. (1997). Explaining Fertility Transition. *Demography*, Vol., 34, No. 4, pp. 443-454.

The study attempts at explaining fertility transitions. It argues that even though there are many theories of fertility transition none provides a complete explanation for all known fertility declines. She puts forward four reasons why this has arisen. One, assuming that all transitions have the same cause. Two, ignoring mortality decline as a precondition of fertility decline. Three, assuming that the regulation of fertility is fundamentally different in pretransitional and posttransitional populations. Four, focusing on a decadal time scale.

040. Montgomery, M.R. & J.B. Casterline. (1996). Social Learning, Social influence, and New Models of Fertility. In: Fertility in the United States: New Patterns, New Theories edited by J. B Casterline, R. D. Lee, & K. A. Foote. *Population and Development Review*, Vol. 22, Suppl, pp. 151-75. New York, New York.

The study describes a model for fertility that contains elements that have been neglected-although often parenthetically acknowledged-in most fertility research. Concepts of social learning and social influence are developed based on insights from several social science disciplines.

041. Notestein, F. (1945). Population-The Long View, in T.P. Schultz (ed.). *Food for the World.* Chicago. University of Chicago Press, pp. 36-57.

The author introduces the demographic transition model, one of the earliest models of fertility change. The main tenets of the model are that industrialisation and concomitant urbanisation are preconditions to fertility transitions.

042. Omran, A.R. (1971). The epidemiologic transition theory: A theory of the epidemiology of population change. *Milbank Memorial Fund Quarterly*, Vol. 49, pp. 6-47.

This study looks at the relevance of the epidemiological transition model in explaining demographic and health transitions. The author argues that epidemiological changes induce shifts in demographic orientations, and that improvements in child survival is a major pre-requisite for sustained fertility decline.

043. Pollak, R. & S. Watkins. (1993). Cultural and economic approaches to fertility: Proper marriage or Mésalliance? *Population and Development Review*, 19 No 3, pp. 467-496

Fertility research has been guided by a number of economic models during the past two decades. Behind these models is the premise that preferences are fixed and those fertility differences can be explained solely by differences in opportunities. But this has not always been so. The evidence of fertility transition appears inconsistent with explanations based solely on differences in opportunities. The study takes up these issues by first addressing the consistency of the empirical findings and the interpretations drawn from various fixed preference economic models. They then go on to discuss variable preference economic models, the roles that diffusion may play in these models, and the relationship between cultural and economic explanations of fertility.

044. Potter, J. E. (1989). Parallels between the Health transition and the Fertility transition. *Health Transition Review*, No 2. Vol. 1, pp. 85-91.

The study looks at the relationship between the health transition and the fertility transition. The thrust of the study is simply that most of the reasons for keeping the two areas of inquiry apart are not good reasons, and that there is considerable overlap and complementality between them.

045. Retherford, R. (1985). A theory of marital fertility transition. *Population Studies* 39, pp. 249-268.

The author develops a theory of marital fertility transition based on birth-control diffusion, mortality decline and economic and social development within a common analytical framework.

046. Riley, A.P., A.I. Hermalin, L. Rosero-Bixby. (1993). A new look at the determinants of non-numeric response to desired family size: The case of Costa Rica. *Demography*, 30, No. 2, pp. 159-174.

This article looks at the concept of desired family size in explaining fertility behaviour and trends. The study argues that respondents who give non-numeric answers to questions on desired family size sometimes indicate preferences in other ways. This could be due to factors such as the characteristics of the respondents, and the mode of eliciting information.

047. Robinson, W. C. (1997). The Economic Theory of fertility over Three Decades. *Population Studies*, 51 (1), pp. 63-74.

The micro economic theory of fertility had a promising start in fertility explanations when it was initially formulated more than 20 years ago. Since then this approach has not had a major impact on fertility decisions or in terms of policy. The author examines this disappointment and looks at the emergence of the now dominant versions of the economic approach dubbed the "Chicago school".

048. Rosero-Bixby, L & J. B. Casterline (1993). Modelling Diffusion effects in fertility transition. *Population Studies,* 47, pp. 147-67.

The study examines the implications of simple mathematical models of fertility transition that contain social interaction diffusion effects. The author's advance the hypothesis that diffusion effects act as a third type of causal agent of fertility transition, above and beyond the traditionally studied demand and supply factors.

049. Smith, H. L. (1989). Integrating theory and research on the institutional determinants of fertility. *Demography,* 26, No 2, pp. 171-184.

The article links recent conceptual theories regarding the determinants of fertility with research designs appropriate for testing these theories. The most important causal factors in these theories, typically social or cultural institutions, are properly conceptualised at the macro level.

050. Stokes, C. (1995). Explaining the demographic transition: Institutional factors in fertility decline. *Rural Sociology.* 60 (1), pp. 1-22.

The study reviews transition theory and argues for the theoretical importance of institutional factors in fertility decline in Sub-Saharan Africa.

051. Szreter, S. (1993). The idea of the demographic transition and the study of fertility change. A Critical Intellectual History. *Population and Development Review*, Vol. 19, No. 4, pp. 659-701.

Based on an historical account of the demographic transition theory, the author calls for a movement away from the transition theory ideals if we are to make further intellectual progress in the study of fertility change.

052. Van de Kaa, D. (1987). Europe's second demographic transition. *Population Bulletin* 42 (1), pp. 3-57.

The author makes mention of a second demographic transition in Europe where fertility declines below replacement levels, which if allowed to continue will lead to population decline.

053. Van de Walle, E. (1992). Fertility transition, conscious choice, and numeracy. *Demography*, Vol. 29, No 4, pp. 487-502.

The author examines the concept of fertility transition and argues that the mentality, which leads to family limitation, includes numeracy about children.

054. Wilson, C., J. Oeppen, & M. Pardoe. (1988). What is natural fertility? The modelling of a concept. *Population Index*, 54, pp. 4-20

The study examines the value of the concept of natural fertility using Coale-Trussel model of marital fertility.

2

Fertility Decline in Latin America

055. Alba, F. & J. E. Potter. (1986). Population and development in Mexico since 1940: An interpretation. *Population and Development Review,* 12, No 1, pp. 47-75.

The rise in the socially perceived need for fertility control to maintain norms in Mexico is examined. The article also traces the post war increase and the decline in Mexican income growth rates.

056. Aramburu, C. (1994). Is Population Policy necessary? Latin America and the Andean Countries. *Population and Development Review*, 1994, 20 (suppl) pp. 159-178.

This article examines the relationship between population policy and demographic change in Latin American countries. It is observed that in countries such as Peru, with explicit population policies often have weak official family planning programs and modest contraceptive prevalence rates, while others like Brazil, which lack a policy commitment to induce fertility decline, show high contraceptive prevalence rates although a very limited method predominates.

057. Barroso, C. (1988). Fertility decline and public policies in Brazil. Paper presented at the American Assembly on US Policy towards World Population Growth. Minneapolis: University of Minnesota.

The influence of public policy on the Brazilian fertility transition is examined.

058. Bravo, J.H. (1992). Theoretical Views of the fertility transition in Latin America: what is the relevance of a diffusionist approach? *Notas de Poblacion,* Vol. 20, No. 56, Dec 1992, 33-55 pages, Santiago, Chile.

The fertility transitions in Latin America are reviewed within the framework of transition theory and the diffusionist perspective. The analysis indicates that the elements of the standard transition theory appear to be useful, but limited in their explanation of the observed declines in the region. The available evidence for the last few decades indicate that, in general, aggregate relations between fertility and development indicators have shifted and become less steep over time.

059. Brems, S. K. (1993). *Caretakers of blood: fertility transition in rural Northeast Brazil.* Ph.D dissertation John Hopkins University. 783 pages.

The dynamics of fertility change in a poor, rural region of Brazil is examined based on both quantitative and qualitative methods. The relationships among fertility and the political economy, traditional beliefs, and social organisation are also explored.

060. Carvalho, J.A, P.D. A. Paiva & D.R. Sawyer. (1981). The recent sharp decline in fertility in Brazil: Economic boom, social inequality and baby bust. *Working Paper, Latin America and Caribbean Regional Office, the Population Council.*

Brazil has recently experienced a sharp fall in fertility. The authors explore the decline in fertility by looking at the respective roles of the economic boom, social inequality and the baby bust.

061. Carvalho, J. A. & L.R. Wong. (1992). Fertility transition in Brazil. *Notas de Poblacion*, Vol. 20, No. 56, Dec. 1992. 107-41 pp. Santiago, Chile.

The authors examine fertility trends in Brazil for the period 1940-1985. Although it followed the processes of socio-economic and industrial development and of urbanisation, the fertility reduction was most pronounced in two periods: 1970-75 and 1980-85. The first period coincides with what has been called the Economic Miracle, which was paradoxically accompanied by indicators of a substantial deterioration in the quality of life of the least favoured socio-economic groups. The second period coincides with the international economic crisis of the 1980s, which has disproportionately affected Brazil, when compared with other Latin American countries, given that it is more industrialised and involved in the international market.

062. Carvalho, J.A. (1993-1994). Population and development-the Brazilian example. *Zeitschrift fur Bevolkerungswissenschaft,* Vol. 19, no. 3 1993-1994. 258-62 pp. Wiesbaden, Germany.

The author explores trends in population and development in Brazil. The peculiar economic, social and demographic evolution of Brazil during the last four decades is an interesting process that reveals both the complexity of the relationship between the economy and population and the rather limited capacity to foresee the path of the demographic dynamics in a country. The study argues that the rapid and generalised fertility decline in Brazil without any governmental policy on population and or birth control can teach us about determinants of fertility transition in a relatively underdeveloped country with huge social and regional inequalities.

063. Chackiel, J. & S. Schkolnik. (1996). Latin America: Overview of the Fertility Transition, 1950-1990. In J.Guzman, S. Singh, G. Rodriguez, E. Pantelides (eds.). *The Fertility Transition in Latin America.* Oxford. Clarendon Press, pp. 3-26.

The study provides an overview of the major trends in fertility change in Latin America between the period 1950 to 1990.

064. Diaz-Briquets, S. & L. Perez. (1982). Fertility decline in Cuba. *Population and Development Review*, Vol. 8, pp. 513-37.

The objective of the paper is to offer a socio-economic interpretation of the Cuban fertility decline taking into account the peculiar nature of Cuban history since 1959, the date that marked the beginning of a revolutionary period that entailed a complete revamping of the nations social and economic structures. While observers have often attributed the fertility decline to modernisation over the last two decades, the authors argue for a more complex explanation in which baby boom and bust arose from objective factors in social and economic trends and subjective factors related to public consumption aspirations and expectations. In this view, the baby boom was a response to the economic achievements and social welfare reforms of the early years of the revolution and the feelings of optimism they engendered in the public. The subsequent dramatic downturn in fertility was a response to deteriorating economic conditions and wide public perception of unmet aspirations as well as modernisation.

065. Dierckxsens, W. (1994). Costa Rica-the unfinished demographic transition. In: *Understanding reproductive change; Kenya, Tamil Nadu, Punjab, Costa Rica,* edited by B. Egero and M. Hammarskjold. 1994. 135-63 pp. Lund University Press, Lund. Sweden.

Costa Rica has experienced a substantial decline in fertility during the last three decades. This study focuses on the links between falling fertility and improvements in social services. Fertility decline was already well underway when in 1968 a national family planning program made possible a rapid diffusion of contraceptive use. During the economic and social crisis of the early 1980s, the fertility transition was temporarily halted. The author analyses differential responses to the crisis, and the impact on childbearing of the subsequent growth of employment in the informal sector.

066. Ebanks, G. E; P. M. George & C. E. Nobbe. (1974). Fertility and Number of

Partnerships in Barbados. *Population Studies,* 28, pp. 449-461.

This article examines patterns of sexual union formation as well as the relationship between these patterns and fertility in the English-speaking Caribbean. The main lessons are that sexual unions in the British Caribbean are unstable and that this instability depresses fertility.

067. Ebanks, G. E; P.M.George; C. E. Nobbe. (1975). Emigration and Fertility Decline: The Case of Barbados. *Demography,* 12 (3). August 1975, pp. 431-45.

The study examines the role of emigration in the fertility declines, which have occurred on the island of Barbados between 1960 and 1970. The discussion suggests that emigration is an important factor in the fertility declines, which have been occurring on the island of Barbados.

068. Ferrando, D. & C. Aramburu. (1992). Fertility transition in Peru. *Notas de Poblacion*, Vol. 20, No. 56, Dec 1992, pp. 173-202. Santiago, Chile.

The fertility transition in Peru is examined, emphasising the differences across socio-cultural groups. Changes in the level and structure of fertility in the Coastal region, the Mountain Range, and the Jungle are compared. Then, the role of nuptiality and contraception in explaining the fertility decline is discussed. In order to better understand the complexity of factors involved in the practice of contraception, some results of a study on attitudes toward sexuality and contraception of women from three generation groups and three cultural contexts are presented.

069. Florez, C.E. (1992). The fertility transition and family urban income distribution in Colombia. *Sociological Inquiry*, vol. 62, No 2, pp. 169-84.

The effect of social and demographic changes on family income distribution in the largest Colombian cities between 1967 and 1968 and 1984 and 1985 are examined. The findings of the study suggest that urban family income distribution worsened showing disparities among the middle income group, the richest and the poorest. The deterioration in urban family income inequality is explained with reference to households with more educated heads, those with working wives and finally those with smaller families and with fewer children.

070. Fort, A.L. (1992). Fertility and reproductive behaviour in Peru: Andes mountains and the Amazon basin. *Estudios Demografiscos y Urbanos,* Vol.7, No.2-3, May-Dec 1992. 327-57, 619 pp. Mexico City, Mexico.

The article attempts to discuss the historical and contemporary situations of fertility among populations residing in the two least studied areas of Peru: the Andes mountains and the Amazon basin. The study starts with a review of the demographic catastrophe that the Spanish presence meant to the people of these areas. The harmful effects of the rubber boom and more recently, of oil boom periods are also reviewed. Fertility trends in the two areas are analysed, with a focus on marriage, breast-feeding, and contraceptive use.

071. Frejka, T. & L.C. Atkin. (1996). The role of induced abortion in the fertility transition of Latin America. In: *The Fertility Transition in Latin America*, edited by Jose M. Guzman, S. Singh, G. Rodriguez, and E. A. Pantelides. Pp. 179-91. Clarendon Press, Oxford.

The study looks at the contributions of induced abortion in the Latin American fertility transition. Model calculations are used to arrive at the relative contribution of induced abortion to fertility control. Given the fact that the desire to limit births exists in the region, the authors argue that people will resort to abortions relatively frequent if efforts are not made to make contraception more accessible and available to the population.

072. Fuller, G. (1974). On the Spatial Diffusion of Fertility Decline: The Distance-to Clinic Variable in a Chilean Community. *Economic Geography,* 50 (4). Oct. pp. 321-32.

The study looks at the relative importance of distance between residence and contraceptive supply as determinants of fertility decline in a Chilean community.

073. Goldani, A.M. (1988). Women's Transitions: The Intersection of Female Life Course, Family and Demographic Transitions in Twentieth Century Brazil. Ph.D. dissertation, University of Texas, Austin.

The thesis explores the fertility decline in Brazil within the context of changes in women's life course transitions.

074. Gomez V. (1989). Fertility Change in Costa Rica: 1964-86. Unpublished Doctoral Dissertation University of Wisconsin.

The thesis explores the changes in fertility in Costa Rica between the period 1964 and 1986.

075. Gonzales-Cortez, G. (1974). *Developmental Measures leading to a Decline in Fertility in Underdeveloped Countries of Latin America. The Cases of Brazil, Chile, and Cuba.* Santiago, Centro Latinoamericano de Demografia. May 1974, 47 pages. Series A, no 120.

This study deals with a wide range of development policies and their possible influences on fertility behaviour. The analysis includes policies in effect in Brazil during the medici government, in Chile under Allende and in Cuba under Castro. Each of the three countries is viewed in terms of its relative structural heterogeneity, a concept that refers to the co-existence within a society of economic and social patterns corresponding to different stages of the development process in more advanced industrial societies.

076. Guzman, J. & J. Rodriguez. (1993). Pre-transitional fertility in Latin America: a forgotten chapter. *Notas de Poblacion*, Vol. 21, No. 57, Jun 1993, pp. 217-46. Santiago, Chile.

Total fertility trends for four Latin American countries, Chile, Costa Rica, Colombia and Honduras are investigated. Calculations show that pre-transitional fertility was not higher than observed at the beginning of its sustained reduction. On the other hand, persistent differences are to be observed between fertility in urban areas and fertility in rural areas. From the levels of certain urban areas it is possible to conclude that as far as the 30s decade, or even before, there existed social groups which limited their offspring. The study concludes that patterns of birth control behaviour were observed long before the 60s decade, at least within certain social groups. Nevertheless, it was only by the mid 60s after a series of structural changes in Latin American societies, that these behaviours had a repercussion on other social strata, thus producing a decrease in average fertility.

077. Guzman, J. (1994). The Onset of Fertility Decline in Latin America. In Therese Locoh (edit). *The Onset of Fertility Transition, in Sub-Saharan Africa,* pp. 43-67 Ordina etc. International Union for the scientific study of Population.

This article focuses on the analysis of the time in which fertility transition began in Latin America. It is observed that in most countries of Latin America a general process of fertility decline began in the sixties. This radical change originated in an important shift in the reproductive behaviour.

078. Guzman, J, S. Singh, G. Rodriguez, & E. A. Pantelides (Eds.) (1996*). The Fertility Transition in Latin America.* Oxford. Clarendon Press 449 pages.

This book grew out of an IUSSP conference in Buenos Aires in April 1990. The book covers 23 chapters on various aspects of the Latin American fertility transition.

079. Haghshenas, H. (1991). *Proletarianization and Fertility: Do the Developing Countries repeat the experience of the European Societies*? Ph.D Dissertation the University of Texas at Austin 263 Pages.

The study explores the relationship between fertility behaviour and the process of social change in the early European experience and in the contemporary developing countries with emphasis on Brazil as a case study. The study emphasises that the protoindustrialization in Europe created conditions conducive to rapid population growth, which changed the life style and the character of the European societies. By contrast empirical analysis of 25 contemporary developing nations in general and Brazil in particular in the 1960s and 1970s indicates that the proletarianization process is incomplete and its impact on fertility has been negative.

080. Handwerker, W.P (1989). *Women's Power and Social Revolution: Fertility Transition in the West Indies.* Newbury Park, California. Sage, 1989, 254 pages.

Based on individual and societal level data derived from Barbados, Handweker underlies the weaknesses of conventional modernisation and westernisation explanations of third world fertility decline, developing in their place a deductive theory that draws on the ideas of Charles Darwin, Karl Marx and Adam Smith.

081. Handwerker, W.P. (1992). West Indian Gender relations, family planning programs and fertility decline. *Social Science and Medicine,* Vol. 35, No. 10. pp. 1245-1257.

Based on data derived from Barbados and Antigua, the author argues that education by itself had no effect on fertility, but that education combined with opportunities for employment had major impacts on fertility decline.

082. Handwerker, W. P. (1993). Empowerment and fertility transition on Antigua, WI: education, employment, and the moral economy of childbearing. *Human Organisation,* Vol. 52, No. 1, spring 1993. 41-52 pages. Oklahoma City, Oklahoma.

The author examines the impact of education and employment opportunities on the fertility transition in Antigua, using data collected in field studies in 1987 and 1989. The results indicate that Antiguan women's birth trajectories are functions of their view of the moral economy of childbearing, which in turn is a function of the conjunction of improved employment opportunities and increased educational attainment. Women's educational attainment, however, is a function of improved employment opportunities. Education by itself had almost nothing to do with Antigua's decline to replacement-level fertility. Education together with expanding employment opportunities had everything to do with it.

083. Hicks, W. W. (1974). Economic Development and Fertility Change in Mexico 1950-1970. *Demography,* pp. 407-422.

The study explores the responses of fertility to economic development and the decline in mortality in Mexico. Factors associated with differences in completed fertility in

1970 in the states of Mexico are analysed, changes in fertility during the period from 1951-1953 to 1969-1971 are established and the concomitant economic factors associated with these changes are also examined. The most important factors acting to reduce TFR over time are increases in life expectancy and declines in the share of the labour force in agriculture. However, these two variables by themselves are not adequate to achieve a rapid decline in fertility in the future.

084. Hogan, D. & C. E. Florez. (1990). Demographic transition and Life Course Change in Columbia. *Journal of Family History*, 15 pp. 1-21.

The Colombian demographic transition is analysed within the framework of changes in the lifecourse patterns.

085. Holl, K.D, G. C. Daily, P.R. Ehrlich. (1993). The fertility plateau in Costa Rica. A review of causes and remedies. *Environment and Conservation*, 20 (4) pp. 317-323.

This article looks at the fertility plateau in Costa Rica. The decline and subsequent above replacement plateau in Costa Rican fertility rates illustrates a demographic pattern that is apparent in other developing countries. This paper discusses the complexity of factors that contribute to the fertility plateau in Costa Rica. These contributory factors include the social and economic status of women, socio-economic conditions in general, lack of government commitment to and supply of family planning services relative to demand, deficient sex and family planning education, and the powerful institutional influence of the catholic church.

086. Hollerbach, P E. & S. Diaz-Briquets (1983). *Fertility Determinants in Cuba*. Committee on Population and Demography Report, No. 26, 1983, 242 pages. NRC, Committee on Population and Demography, Washington, D.C.

This report is one of a series of country studies of fertility determinants sponsored by the Committee on Population and Demography, National Research Council of the USA. Demographic trends in Cuba are analysed for the period before and after the revolution of 1959. The proximate determinants of fertility are also discussed.

087. Inter-American Development Bank. (1993). *Latin America in Graphs: Demographic and Economic Trends, 1972-1992*. 2nd ed. 200 pages. Washington, D.C. Distributed by John Hopkins University Press, Baltimore, MD.

This book provides a graphical illustration of population trends in Latin America for the 26 developing member countries of the Inter-American Development Bank (IDB), for Latin America as a region and for four main economic regions: Andean Pact, CACM, CARICOM and MERCOSUR based on the United Nations medium variant projections. Standard graphs are provided on major demographic and economic trends in Latin America. Major topics include: population and vital statistics, labour force, national accounts, balance of payments, external trade by destination and origin and external debt.

088. James, W.H. (1966). The effect of altitude on fertility in Indean Countries. *Population Studies*, Vol. Xx, No 1.

In papers previously published in the Population Studies Journal, J.Y Stycos and D.M. Heer have shown that fertility is lower in the economically underdeveloped Indian speaking parts of Peru, Ecuador and Bolivia than in the more prosperous Spanish-speaking parts. Stycos concluded that the reason for the fertility difference in Peru is the greater marital instability of the Indian speakers, which decreased their total exposure to the risk of conception. Heer suggested instead that the causes of the difference might be voluntary. The present paper questions Heer's analysis and offers the explanation that the difference may be attributed to the physiological effects of altitude.

089. Jones, W.R. (1977). Fertility Decline in Barbados. Some Spatial Considerations. *Studies in Family Planning,* Vol. 8, No. 6, pp. 157-163.

The study uses areal analysis in examining the factors affecting fertility within the Barbados context. The findings of the study reveal that a concentration of family planning programs in areas of greatest accessibility and modernisation contributes to spatial variations in fertility.

090. Juarez, F & S. Llera. (1996). The process of family formation during the fertility transition. In. *The fertility transition in Latin America,* (ed.). By J. Guzman, S. Singh, G. Rodriguez, and E. A. Pantelides, pp. 48-73. Clarendon Press Oxford.

This study examines the similarities and dissimilarities in the family formation process in various Latin American countries undergoing the transition to lower levels of fertility. The data are from the WFS and the DHS surveys in Brazil, Colombia, the Dominican Republic, Ecuador and Peru. A brief description of changes in general levels of fertility in Latin America is given in the first section, the next section contains details of variations in the family formation process over the past ten years among several countries of the region, then a general review of family patterns in 1986-87 (inter-country analysis) is given, and finally, evidence is presented on certain variables that intervene in the process of change.

091. Kaufman, G. (1991). *Family formation and fertility in a favela in Belo Horizonte, Brazil: an analysis of cultural and demographic influences*. D.Phil. thesis, Oxford University.

The study looks at demographic and cultural influences on fertility in a *favela* in Brazil.

092. Kaufmann, G. (1993). Family Planning in urban Brazil: gaps between policy and practice. *IDS Discussion Paper* No. 329. Brighton: Institute of Development Studies.

Brazil has experienced a rapid decline in fertility over the last 30 years with little government intervention. This article examines the links between the actual use of contraceptive methods in a *favela,* in Belo Horizonte, and government family planning policy and provision. It is argued that the government should not range against sterilisation but provide it as an answer to the voices of the poor urban women.

093. Klijzing, F. & H. Taylor. (1982). Spatial order in the Demographic Transition: The Costa Rican Case. *Revista Geografica,* 96, pp. 54-59.

The dynamics of the Costa Rican demographic transition is examined with special emphasis on its spatial dimensions.

094. Lam, D.G.S. & S. Duryea. (1993). Increases in education and fertility decline in Brazil. Paper presented at the Annual meeting of the Population Association of America.

The Brazilian fertility decline is examined within the context of increases in education.

095. Le Vine, R.A, Le Vine, S. E., Richman, A., Tapia, U.F.M., Correa, C.S., Muller, P.M. (1991). Women's schooling and child care in the demographic transition: a Mexican case study. *Population and Development Review,* Vol. 17, no. 3, pp. 459-496.

The question of how female school attendances influence fertility and child survival was studied by the authors at the community level in one urban and one rural setting in central Mexico. Maternal schooling was found to be a significant predictor of reductions in fertility and the risks to child's survival in both settings after having controlled for household socio-economic factors.

096. Loyola, M.A. (1993). Infant mortality, fertility, and social institutions. In International Population Conference: Montreal, 1993, Volume 1. 1993. pp 65-72. International Union for the Scientific Study of Population (IUSSP), Liege, Belgium.

The role of social institutions in the decline in fertility and infant mortality in Latin America is analysed based on evidence from the city of Parnaba, Brazil.

097. Manatou, J M. (ed.) (1982). *The Demographic Revolution in Mexico 1970-1980.* Mexico. Mexican Institute of Social Security 1982, 500 pages.

This book provides a thorough overview and description of the history of Mexican population policy and the national plan for family planning and offers a rich analysis of demographic trends and survey data in Mexico during its recent period of sharp fertility decline.

098. Martine, G. (1996). Brazil's fertility decline, 1965-95: A Fresh Look at Key Factors. *Population and Development Review*, 22 (1), pp. 47-75.

This article looks at a variety of factors that underlie Brazil's rapid fertility decline between the period 1965 to 1995. It is argued that the decline took place during a period of both rapid economic growth and economic crisis. The institutional changes introduced by the military government in the 1960s also had an impact on birth control. Some of the institutional factors include health and social security. Other factors of note include the strong influence of the mass media.

099. Merrick, T. & D. H. Graham. (1979). *Population and Economic Development in Brazil: 1800 to the Present.* The John Hopkins University Press, 1979, 385 pages.

The book follows two well defined but interrelated lines of investigation. After providing historical overviews of Brazilian economy and population growth, the authors first address the format, growth, absorption and redistribution of the labour force. They cover the demographics of slavery and European migration during the coffee export phase of Brazilian economic history, long run changes in spatial distribution and in the growth and structure of the labour force, and more recent issues such as urban growth, internal migration, and urban poverty. The second focus of the volume is on fertility and mortality trends and their interrelations with economic development. With regards to fertility trends the authors question whether a transition from higher to lower fertility is underway. They note that the observable fertility decline is typically an urban phenomenon of the more developed regions.

100. Merrick, T. & E. Berquo. (1983). *The Determinants of Brazils' Recent Rapid Decline in Fertility.* Committee on Population and Demography Report. Washington, D.C: National Academy Of Science Press.

The study provides a detailed discussion of the rapid decline in fertility in Brazil looking at trends in fertility as well as explanations underlying the decline in fertility.

101. Merrick, T. (ed.). (1991). Population Pressures in Latin America. *Population Bulletin*, Vol. 41, 350 pages.

The bulletin provides a concise account of population issues in Latin America looking at major demographic trends between 1950 to 1985. It touches on several aspects of the Latin American demography including mortality decline, fertility trends and differentials, marriage and family structure, urban and rural populations, work and education, international migration, population growth and development, population policy as well as future population prospects.

102. Moreno, L. & S. Singh (1996). Fertility decline and changes in proximate determinants in the Latin America and Caribbean regions. In J.M. Guzman et. al. (Eds.). *The Fertility transition in Latin America.* Oxford University Press pp. 113-134.

The study examines the contributions of the proximate determinants to fertility decline in Latin America. The study demonstrates that increasing use of contraception played a major role in the decline.

103. Moreno, L. (1990). Changes in marital fertility in Mexico: Results of two models. *Notas de Poblacion,* Vol. 18, No 50, pp. 75-92.

Two models of marital fertility namely the Coale-Trussel and Rodriguez-Cleland are used to analyse the changes in marital fertility in Mexico between the mid 1970s and the mid 1980s. The data is drawn from World Fertility Survey and the Demographic and Health Surveys Programmes. The study concludes that it is insufficient to interpret the Mexican fertility transition as the passage from a natural state to a controlled one, given that volitional practices for birth spacing seem to have existed before the implementation of family planning programmes was even considered in Mexico.

104. Mundigo, A. (1996). The role of family planning programmes in the fertility transition of Latin America. In Gutzmans et. al. (Eds.). *The fertility Transition in Latin America,* pp. 192-210. Oxford University Press.

The author reviews the role of family planning programs in the Latin American fertility transition and concludes that they were facilitators of the mass transition rather than the agents responsible for these changes. The study is based on data collected during the 1960s and 1970s on abortion and more recently on fertility and contraception prevalence.

105. Noble, J. & M. Potts (1996). The fertility transition in Cuba and the Federal Republic of Korea. The impact of organised family planning. *Journal of Biosocial Science,* 28, pp. 211-225.

The study examines the effects of family planning on fertility decline in Korea and

Cuba. It concludes that access to contraception; voluntary sterilisation and safe abortion have a direct impact on fertility and has been associated with a rapid fall in family size in the two different countries.

106. Oechsli, F.W. & D. Kirk (1975). Modernisation and the Demographic Transition in Latin America and the Caribbean. *Economic Development and Cultural Change*, 23 (3), pp. 391-419.

The study looks at the effects of modernisation on demographic change in Latin America and the Caribbean. It argues that not only is the demographic change speeded up, development and modernisation processes, which include demographic change, have become more rapid.

107. Palloni, A; K. Hill; G, Pinto; A, Guirre. (1996). Economic Savings and Demographic Changes in the History of Latin America. *Population Studies* 50, pp. 105-132.

This article looks at the effects of short-term fluctuations in indicators of economic well being on selected demographic variables such as births, marriage and deaths at age intervals in eleven Latin American countries between 1910 and 1990. The study uses conventional distributed lag models to assess the magnitude and direction of effect and test a variety of hypotheses some of which have been posed to hold in Western Europe and others are more specific and tailored to the Latin American context. It also compares the magnitude and direction of effects obtained among these countries with those obtained for pre-industrial Europe and uncovers the existence of broadly similar patterns.

108. Pantelides, E. (1992). More than a century of Argentine fertility: its evolution since 1869. *Notas de Poblacion,* Vol.20, No.56, Dec 1992, pp. 87-106. Santiago, Chile.

The study provides a descriptive review of the process underling the Argentine fertility decline. Special attention is paid to the period of initiation of the fertility descent in the years following 1895. The study argues that the massive arrival of foreigners coming from countries with lower fertility rates than those prevailing in Argentina had a depressing effect on fertility levels. Additionally, this variable combined with local factors such as the progressive concentration of population in areas of lower fertility specifically urban areas. Finally, the study ends in the decade of the 1970s, noting the explosion of births, and the conclusion is reached here that one is dealing with a genuine increase of cohort completed fertility.

109. Parrado, E.A & M. Tienda. (1997). Women's Roles and Family Formation in Venezuela. New Forms of Consensual Unions? *Social Biology,* Vol. 44, No. 1-2 pp. 1-24.

This paper assesses the effects of changes in women's education and labour force participation on nuptiality patterns and their implications for fertility decline in Venezuela. Results show that together with delays in union formation, changes in women's education and labour force participation produced a different, more modern type of consensual union, which coexists with traditional consensual unions. Traditional consensual unions remain a substitute for formal marriage among women from rural origins with low levels of education and higher levels of work experience. The study argues that modern consensual unions appear to be an option for well-educated women of urban origins. As in developed countries, these unions assume the form of a trial period before marriage or an alternative to singlehood. Modern consensual unions are unstable than traditional consensual unions and they are associated with lower fertility.

110. Pillet, B.D. (1980). *Fertility Changes in the Early Decades of rapid Socio-economic Development: A Statistical Description of the recent Mexican experience.* Ph.D. Dissertation Stanford University 487 pages.

Using data from Mexico, the author explores the relation of fertility to socio-economic development in Mexico from 1950 to 1970. The study revealed similarity in determinants of fertility for rural and urban localities, as well as significant demographic constraints in the cities, and negative influence on fertility from the following: urbanisation, nonreligious affiliation, indigenous background, low level of living, and female employment and education.

111. Population Reference Bureau. (PRB) (1992). *Fertility & Family Planning in Latin America: Challenges of the 1990s.* Population Reference Bureau.

This book provides information on fertility levels and trends in Latin American countries from 1960 to 1990. It shows that the timing and pace of fertility declines has varied in different countries within the period. Fertility in rural areas is consistently higher and has declined more slowly than fertility in urban areas.

112. Potter, J.E, G. M. Ordonez, A. R. Measham. (1976). The rapid decline in Colombian Fertility. *Population and Development Review,* 2, no. 3/4. pp. 509-531.

Data from the 1973 Colombian census and information from other sources are used to establish an estimate of the current level of national fertility. Comparing this estimate with others for earlier periods indicates that Colombia is moving through a fertility transition that is about as rapid as any on record. It strongly suggests that the availability of modern contraceptive methods increased in response to an emerging demand for fertility limitation generated by general socio-economic development.

113. Prada-Salas, E. (1996). The fertility transition and adolescent childbearing: the case of Colombia. In: *The fertility transition in Latin America,* (ed.). By J. Guzman, S. Singh, G. Rodriguez, and E. Pantelides, pp. 310-22. Clarendon Press, Oxford, England.

The aim of this study is to examine the recent fertility behaviour of adolescents during the years of Colombia's demographic transition, especially in terms of educational levels, the consequences of early childbearing, the country's present situation compared with that of others in the Latin American region, and a possible future course of action for the coming years. Data are primarily taken from the 1986 Colombia Demographic and Health Survey.

114. Rios, R. (1991). Economic development and family size. *American Economist,* Vol.35, No.2, fall 1991. 81-5 pp. New York, New York.

The Latin American demographic transition is compared with that of Europe. The author observes that the fall in mortality in Latin America has failed to lower family size. He finds this result as not theoretically sound as reduced mortality makes children cheaper and is expected to reduce fertility but to increase the number of survivors. Development and modernisation encourages family limitation in Western Europe, changes similar in nature have attended the mortality decline in Latin America, but often these changes have been modest in size. The author observed that deviations from the Western European transition follow a pattern: least developed countries deviate the most, while most developed countries deviate the least.

115. Rodriguez, G. (1992). Spacing and limiting components of the fertility transition in Latin America. *Notas de Poblacion,* Vol.20, No.56, Dec 1992. 57-86 pp. Santiago, Chile.

This study looks at marital fertility within categories of three socio-economic factors: residence, wives' education and husbands' occupation, for the six Latin American countries which have participated both in the World Fertility Survey (WFS) and Demographic and Health Surveys (DHS) program. A statistical model of the period marital fertility of individual women is used which permits a succinct description of levels and patterns of fertility by age and duration of union, and yields estimates of indices of spacing and control. The study concludes that despite the diversity of conditions in the region, the indices of spacing and control in different social strata appear to have followed a common path of increase over time, which is shown to be consistent with a simple mathematical model of social diffusion.

116. Rodriguez, G. (1996). The spacing and limiting components of the fertility transition in Latin America. In: *The Fertility transition in Latin America* edited by J. Guzman, S. Singh, G. Rodriguez, and E. Pantelides. pp 127-47. Clarendon Press

Oxford. England.

The study presents the findings on the analysis of marital fertility within categories of key socio-economic factors based on material from six Latin American countries namely, Colombia, Dominican Republic, Ecuador, Mexico, Peru and Trinidad and Tobago.

117. Rosero-Bixby, L. (1991). *Interaction Diffusion and fertility transition in Costa Rica*. Ph.D. Dissertation University of Michigan Ann Arbor. 279 pages.

This study looks at the spread of birth control by social interaction and its influence on fertility in Costa Rica.

118. Rosero-Bixby, L. & J. B. Casterline. (1994). Interaction diffusion and fertility transition in Costa Rica. *Social Forces,* Dec. 73 (2), pp. 435-462.

Based on a dynamic regression model derived from pooled time series data for 100 counties in Costa Rica, the authors demonstrate that information and values through social interaction shaped the timing and pace of the transition from high to low fertility levels in Costa Rica.

119. Rosero-Bixby, L. (1996). Nuptiality trends and fertility transition in Latin America. In Jose M. Guzman et al. (Eds.). *The Fertility transition in Latin America*. Clarendon Press, Oxford.

The study argues that changes in nuptiality patterns appear to have played a trivial role in the fertility transition for the region as a whole, despite significant variation across countries.

120. Rosero-Bixby, L. & J.B. Casterline. (1995). Diffusion through social interaction and fertility transition: quantitative and qualitative evidence from Costa Rica. *Notas de Poblacion*, Vol. 23, No 61, pp. 29-78.

The study adds a new theoretical dimension to the Costa Rican fertility transition by examining the influence of social interaction. The results of the study reveal an ordered spatial pattern suggestive of contagion between neighbouring areas.

121. Seiver, D. A. (1975). Recent fertility in Mexico. Measurement and Interpretation. *Population Studies,* 29, 3, pp. 341-354.

Mexican fertility has remained high in spite of rapid economic development and its concomitants. In order to shed light on the Mexican puzzle of a high birth rate coexisting with rapid economic development, this paper examines the following two questions. Are aggregate fertility measures making a decline in age-specific or region-specific fertility, and if fertility has not declined, can we interprete this phenomenon by explaining cross sectional variations in fertility, which exist in terms of the demographic variables.

122. Silva, N.V; M.H. Henriques, & A. Souza. (1990). An analysis of reproductive behaviour in Brazil. *Demographic and Health Survey: Further Analysis Series*, No.6.

The study identifies two main socio-cultural factors through which modernisation affects fertility, wife's education and her religiosity, both of which indicate the importance of ideational change in the process of fertility transition.

123. Singh, S. & G. Sedgh, (1997). The Relationship of Abortion to Trends in Contraception and Fertility in Brazil, Colombia and Mexico. *International Family Planning Perspectives* Vol. 23, No. 1, pp. 4-14.

The study examines among other things the role of contraceptive use and abortion in accounting for fertility levels and changes in fertility rate in Brazil, Colombia and Mexico. The findings of the study show that the role of abortion to fertility decline was greatly felt in Brazil.

124. Stephen, L.S & R. E. Bilsborrow. (1974). The Barbados Family Planning Association and Fertility Decline in Barbados. *Studies in Family Planning*, Vol. 5, No 10, pp. 325-332.

The author's examine the role of the Barbados family planning programme in the decline in fertility in the country.

125. Studies in Family Planning. (1996). Haiti 1994-1995. Results from the Demographic and Health Survey. *Studies in Family Planning,* 27 (4), pp. 232-236.

This issue of Studies in Family Planning Journal summarises the results of the most recent DHS on Haiti. The analysis is based on interviews carried out among 5356 women aged 15-49 and a subsample of 1610 men aged 15-59. The interviews took place from July 1994 to January 1995. The summary statistics presented cover fertility trends and preferenes, contraceptive use, postpartum variables, infant mortality, health-disease, prevention and treatment, and nutritional status of children younger than 5 years.

126. Stycos J.M. (1978). *Patterns of Fertility Decline in Costa Rica.* International

Population Program, Cornell University, 1978. 193 pages.

This monograph consists of two parts, the decline of fertility in Costa Rica and a pretest of psychological items related to family planning and fertility. The first part focuses on fertility decline from 1961 to 1973, a period in which the crude birth rate declined by 40 percent and the gross reproductive rate by 46 percent. Stycos concludes that changes in age structure and in marriage patterns did not have much effect on fertility changes, but rather that the fertility decline in Costa Rica was initiated and to a considerable extent realised, by young married women.

127. Stycos, J.M. (1982). The Decline of Fertility in Costa Rica: Literacy, Modernisation, and Family Planning. *Population Studies* 36, pp. 15-30.

The study examines the role of literacy, modernisation and family planning in the decline in fertility in Costa Rica.

128. Taylor, A. (1995). Debt, dependence and the demographic transition. Latin America into the next century. *World Development* 23, No 5, pp. 869-879.

The Latin American demographic transition is examined within the context of the debt and dependency burdens.

129. Torrez, P.H. (1996). Bolivia: the social and geographic context of trends in fertility. In: *The Fertility transition in Latin America,* edited by Jose M. Guzman, S. Singh, G. Rodriguez, and E. Pantelides, pp. 359-72 Clarendon Press, Oxford, England.

Patterns of fertility in Bolivia are analysed over the past 15 to 20 years using data from the 1976 census and recent surveys including the 1989 National Demographic and Health Surveys. The author concludes that although overall fertility declined in the 12 to 15 years before 1988, this decline was confined to urban areas, fertility remained high in rural areas, and in some cases actually increased in response to high rates of infant mortality. The author also notes that Bolivia's extreme differences in income distribution are associated with differentials in fertility, and that fertility levels, particularly among the poor are likely to remain high while these inequalities persist.

130. Tung, S. L. (1984). The rapid fertility decline in Guam natives. *Journal of Biosocial Science*, April 16 (2), pp. 231-239.

The author explores the decline in fertility in Guam and the possible factors underlying the decline in fertility.

131. United Nations. Department for Economic and Social Information and Policy

Analysis (1993). *Fertility transition and women's life course in Mexico.* 62 pages. New York, New York.

This report is part of an ongoing program of research on the relationship between the status of women and fertility. The study is one in a series of three, and concerns Mexico. Sources of information are from the Mexican Fertility Survey of 1976-1977, and the National Fertility and Health Survey of 1987. Chapter I provides a review the concepts underlying the study, the methods used and the materials on which it is based. The demographic and background characteristics of the study population are described in chapter II. Chapters III-VI are devoted to the analysis of nuptiality, fertility, labour force participation and living arrangements respectively. A summary of the main findings and some final considerations are presented in chapter VII.

132. United Nations (1993). Centro Latinamericano de Demografia (CELADE) (Santiago, Chile). Latin America: age specific fertility rates, 1950-2025. *Boletin Demografico/Demographic Bulletin*, Vol.36, No.52, Jul 1993. 124 pages. Santiago, Chile.

This demographic bulletin provides data on projections of fertility in Latin America. Following an initial section covering the entire region for the period 1950-2025, data are provided separately by country on estimated and projected fertility rates and structures, according to various hypotheses concerning changes in fertility.

133. Uthoff, A. & G. Gonzalez. (1976). *Women's Participation in Economic Activity a Strategic Factor of Change in Fertility. The Cases of Mexico and Costa Rica.* Geneva, Switzerland, International Labour Office, 1976. 96 pages.

Both Costa Rica and Mexico experienced rapid declines in mortality from 1940 onward but by 1970 Costa Rica's birth rate was much lower than that of Mexico. The authors use census samples of Mexico for 1960 and 1970 and of Costa Rica for 1963 and 1973 to explore the variations in women's participation in economic activity as a factor in explaining the difference in reproductive behaviour.

134. Van Rompaey, S.E. (1993). *The decline of Chilean fertility, 1960-1982: a contextual and multilevel analysis.* Ph.D dissertation, Stanford University. 105 pages.

The study uses national census data for the periods 1960, 1970 and 1982 in developing a series of models to test the relative influence of women's status, socio-economic conditions, and cultural variables on fertility changes in Chile. The findings lend credence to the importance of rural-urban residence on fertility differentials especially as higher women's status is associated with urban residence.

135. Verdugo, L.A. (1994). Marital fertility in Brazil: differential by type of union

and its importance in the fertility transition, 1976-1991. *DHS Working Paper* No. 15, Macro International Demographic and Health Surveys, Calverton, Maryland. Aug 1994. 17 pages.

This paper examines marital fertility differentials in Brazil by type of union during three periods of the fertility transition, 1976, 1984 and 1991. Three regions are covered, the Northeast, Sao Paulo and the South. Levels of education and place of residence are also considered as important covariates in the analysis. The data used in this project originated in the national household surveys.

136. Weinberger, M. B. (1996). Changes in the mix of contraceptive methods during the fertility decline. In: *The fertility transition in Latin America.* Edited by J. Guzman, S. Singh, and G. Rodriguez & E. Pantelides, pp. 151-78.

The author examines changes in the methods of contraception chosen by contraceptive users in Latin America, including the Caribbean. The study argues that the growing use of contraception has been the main proximate cause of the fertility decline that has occurred in recent years. The discussion begins with an overview of contraceptive practice in Latin America as compared with other major regions. After a brief look at trends in the overall level of contraceptive use in Latin America and Caribbean countries, the book examines changes over time in the use of specific contraceptive methods. Finally, for six countries, trends in the use of female sterilisation are examined in more detail drawing on DHS data.

137. White, M.J., L. Moreno & S. Guo. (1991). The Interrelation of fertility and Geographic mobility in Peru: A Hazards Model Analysis. *Population Studies and Training Center (PSTC) Working Paper Series,* Sept. 5, 1991, 34 pages.

The study examines the effect of place of residence and migration on fertility in Peru based on the Peruvian Demographic and Health Survey. The findings of study show that residence in a city (vs countryside) predicts lower fertility but residence in an intermediate size town has no effect.

138. Zavala de Cosio. (1992). The demographic transition in Latin America and Europe. *Notas de Publacion,* Vol.20, No.56, Dec 1992. 11-32, pp. Santiago, Chile.

Two demographic transition models for Latin America are examined in this study. The first is similar to Europe's modern reproductive patterns. The other applies to women with traditional reproductive behaviours, including early marriage and high fertility. The implications of each model for future fertility decline and economic growth are discussed.

139. Zlotnik, H. (1982). *Levels and Recent Trends in Fertility and Mortality in*

Colombia. Washington, D.C. National Academy Press, 1982, 214 pages.

This study sponsored by the Committee on Population and Demography applies a range of sophisticated demographic methods to a variety of Colombian data sets in order to derive the best estimates of levels and recent trends in fertility and mortality. The study concludes that infant mortality in Colombia declined by approximately 40 percent between 1950 and 1960 from a level of 150 deaths per 1000 live births to 85 for both sexes combined and declined by a further 28 percent between 1964 and 1978. Fertility remained fairly constant up to 1964 or 1965, with a total fertility rate of 6.6 or 6.8 children per woman. The decline thereafter has been modelled by a simple linear trend with the total fertility rate falling to 5.1-5.2 children per woman in 1973, 6.4 in 1976 and 4.2 by 1978.

3

Fertility Decline in Asia

140. Adlakha, A. L. & J. Banister (1995). Demographic Perspectives on China and India. *Journal of Biosocial Science,* 27, pp. 163-178.

This article compares levels and trends of population growth rates, age and sex composition, mortality and fertility including family planning practices in the Worlds two most populous countries, China and India. Both countries are undergoing demographic transition but China is nearer than India to achieving a stationary population. Fertility in China has declined below replacement level while in India it is nearly one and half children per woman above replacement level. Both countries have achieved large reductions in mortality but life expectancy at birth in China is currently about 10 years longer than in India. Both countries have young populations but China will proceed India in the ageing of population structure during the 21st century.

141. Aghajanian, A. (1991). Population change in Iran, 1966-86: A stalled demographic transition? *Population and Development Review,* 17, No. 4, pp. 703-715.

The author assesses recent demographic changes in Iran against the background of two sharply different ideological and socio-economic environments, approximated by contrasting the two ten-year periods 1966-76 and 1976-86.

142. Amin, R., J. Chowdhury, M. Kabir, R. Hill. (1994). Recent evidence on trends and differentials in Bangladesh fertility: an update. *Journal of Biosocial Science*, Vol. 26, No 2, pp. 235-41.

A comparison of contraceptive and fertility data for 1985-1991 with data for 1983 shows that fertility has continued to decline in Bangladesh, in all segments of society.

The magnitude of decline varied according to educational level, region and urban-rural locality. The percentage decline in total marital fertility rate was somewhat higher among urban than rural residents, educated women showed greater declines than uneducated, increasing the overall educational differences in total fertility by 1991. Factors contributing to the recent decline in fertility are discussed.

143. ANON. (1990). Asia's demographic future. The next 20 years. *Asia Pacific Population and Policy*, 14, 4 pages.

The study argues that although most countries in Asia have experienced fertility declines, unless fertility falls further, projected population trends are likely to have serious adverse effects in the next twenty years. Rapid population growth in urban areas poses problems for housing, transportation and polution control, while population growth in rural areas is likely to further raise agricultural densities, retarding labour productivity and income growth. The article argues that the most effective programmes for bringing about fertility decline are family planning, maternal and child health and improvements in the status of women.

144. ANON. (1991). Economic development and fertility decline: Lessons from Asia's newly industrialised countries. *Asia Pacific Population and Policy*.

Hong Kong, Korea, Singapore and Taiwan all represent "success stories" in family planning, as well as examples of success in economic growth. The lesson of their success is that development planning and family planning can work closely together to reduce fertility rates.

145. Axelrod, P. (1990). Cultural and Historical factors in the population decline of the Parsis of India. *Population Studies,* 44, pp. 401-419.

The author provides an account of how cultural factors led to fertility decline among the Parsis of India. He links this to a set of values that can be considered as a logical extension of adaptive strategies developed by the Parsis as a minority group in India. The Parsis as a group choose to delay marriages, remain celibate and have fewer children in order to achieve goals that are specific to their community.

146. Axinn, W.G. (1990). *Social change, family organization and fertility limitation: Tests of a theoretical model among the Tamang of Nepal.* Unpublished Ph.D. dissertation, University of Michigan.

The fertility transition among the Tamang of Nepal is analysed based on the influences of social change and family organisation.

147. Axinn, W.G. (1992). Rural Income-generating Programs and Fertility

limitations: Evidence from a Micro-demographic Study in Nepal. *Rural Sociology* 57(3), pp. 396-413.

The study examines the role of rural income-generating programs on fertility decline in Nepal. The findings of the study show that participation in rural development programs increases contraceptive use thereby reducing fertility. The study also shows that program participants are more likely to use contraceptives to limit fertility than non-participants.

148. Axinn, W.G. (1992). Family organisation and fertility limitation in Nepal. *Demography,* 29, (4) 50, pp. 3-21.

The study uses the family mode of organisation framework to link together hypotheses relating social change to fertility limitation. Experiences in non-family activities are predicted to affect fertility behaviour, with the outcome dependent on social, economic, and cultural context. To provide individual level tests of hypotheses the paper uses data from a Nepalese community, which recently began dramatic family and fertility transitions. The findings show that experiences in non-family activities before marriage increase the odds of subsequently adopting fertility limitation in this setting. The evidence also demonstrates the importance of including measures of husband's experiences in models of fertility decisions.

149. Axinn, W.G. (1993). The effects of children's schooling on fertility limitation. *Population Studies,* Vol. 47, No.3, Nov.1993, pp. 481-93.

Many theories of fertility predict that mass education reduces fertility, but this effect may be produced in variety of ways. In this paper, microdemographic data from a rural community in Nepal, in which the spread of mass education and fertility limitation is just beginning are used to examine these links. The analyses contrast the influence of parents and children's educational experiences on parents' fertility preferences and behaviour. The results indicate that children's schooling has a strong influence on both fertility preferences and behaviour. The effects of parental schooling are weaker and also inconsistent in different models. These findings provide support for theories that link mass education to the onset of fertility limitation through children's schooling experience.

150. Backhaus, T., P.B. Belden, T.J. Espenshade. (1994). AIDS, low birth rates, and future growth in Thailand. *Population Today,* Vol. 22, No. 10, Oct 1994. 4-5 pages. Washington, D.C.

The author's examine the demographic impact of the AIDS epidemic on a country with relatively low fertility, using Thailand as an example. They present a range of population scenarios up to the year 2015 depending on the severity of the epidemic.

The results suggest that the AIDS epidemic could have a major impact on future population growth rates in countries with lower fertility levels.

151. Balasubramanian, K. (1992). Emergence of fertility differentials as evidence of fertility decline in India. *Artha Vijnana,* Vol. 34, No 2. June 1992 pp. 182-99, Pune, India.

A review of major studies on fertility concludes that it is only from the late 1960s that movement from the stage of uncontrolled fertility to the stage of controlled fertility leading to the emergence of socio-economic differentials in fertility seems to have really gotten underway in India. This process appears to have been accelerated during the 1970s and 1980s.

152. Bose, A. (1996). Demographic transition and demographic imbalance in India. *Health Transition Review,* Supplement to Volume 6, pp. 89-99.

The study uses data based on the 1991 Census and National Family Health Survey (1992-1993) to highlight the importance of the North-South Demographic Divide in India and its implications for planners and policy makers.

153. Cain, M. (1981). Risk and Insurance. Perspectives on Fertility and Agrarian Change in India and Bangladesh. *Population and Development Review*, 7, No. 3, pp. 435-474.

The author explores fertility responses to risk within the context of rural populations of India and Bangladesh. Maharashtra has one of the lowest fertility rates among all states in India, and there is evidence of declines in fertility in both Maharashtra and Andhra Pradesh.The study argues that in India the diffusion of risk has permitted the relative costliness of children to emerge as an inducement toward smaller sized families. By contrast, Bangladesh has one of the highest and most unyielding fertility rates in all of South Asia. The very high levels of risk in the Bangladesh setting, the role of children in preventing property loss, and the lack of alternative forms of insurance combine to create a powerful disincentive to the adoption of birth control methods.

154. Caldwell, B. (1996). The family and demographic change in Sri Lanka. *Health Transition Review Supplement*, 6, pp. 45-60.

The study looks at how differences in family structure have shaped the demographic regime in Sri Lanka.

155. Caldwell, J.C., P.H. Reddy, & P. Caldwell. (1988). *The Causes of Demographic Change. Experimental Research in South India.* Madison. University

of Wisconsin Press.

Based on a demographic study conducted in the district of Mysore, India between 1979-80, the study argues that family planning programs affected both the desires to have smaller families and the adoption of contraception to achieve this goal.

156. Caldwell, J.C & P. Caldwell. (1992). What does the Matlab fertility experience really show? *Studies in Family Planning,* 23, 5, pp. 292-310.

The family planning program in the Matlab District of Bangladesh has been described in unique detail for more than 25 years and is regarded as a model for equally poor parts of the world. While it is agreed that the Matlab demonstration has been of central importance in showing that fertility can be reduced in Bangladesh, it is argued that many developing countries can draw on this experience to provide less costly family planning programs with less emphasis on the managerial, top down approach.

157. Campbell, B.O., A. Mason, E.M. Pernia. (1993). *The economic impact of demographic change in Thailand, 1980-2015: an application of the HOMES household forecasting model.* 357 pp. East-West Center, Honolulu, Hawaii. Asian Development Bank, Manila, Philippines.

This report summarises demographic trends, household projections, and substantive findings from six studies undertaken as part of a project, Demographic and Economic Forecasting Pilot Study for Thailand, organised and funded by the Asian Development Bank. The purpose of the project was to provide a household projections package, HOMES, to the National Economic and Social Development Board and the National Statistical Office of Thailand, to train staff to use the package, and to explore the ways in which detailed household projections can be used to improve economic forecasting and planning.

158. Casterline, J.B. (1994). Fertility Transition in Asia. In Locoh T. and V. Hertrich (Eds.). *The Onset of Fertility Transition in Sub-Saharan Africa.* pp 69-86. International Union for the Scientific Study of Population.

The study looks at the decline in fertility in Asian countries and the factors underlying these declines. Data is derived from the United Nations, the World Bank, and other International agencies. The study attributes the declines in fertility chiefly to the use of modern contraceptives by married couples. It is argued that the underlying motivation for fertility decline in Asia has been the conviction that children have become costly in economic terms.

159. Chayovan, N; J. Knodel; P. Kamuansilpa. (1988). Approaching Replacement Fertility in Thailand: Results of the 1987 Demographic and Health Survey.

International Family Planning Perspectives, 14, No 3 pp 86-93.

Evidence from the 1987 Thailand Demographic and Health Survey is used to assess the extent of fertility decline in Thailand. The most striking finding is the very low level of recent fertility. For the 24-month period preceding the survey, the total fertility rate of 2.2 is approximately at the replacement level.

160. Cho, L. & K. Kobayashi, (eds.). (1979). *Fertility Transition of the East Asian Population.* Honolulu, The University Press of Hawaii.300 pages.

This book focuses on East Asian countries influenced by Chinese culture that are rapidly experiencing or have completed fertility transition. Japan the Republic of Korea, Singapore, Hong Kong, Malaysia, Taiwan, Thailand, and China. The 13 chapters include revised versions of papers presented at the 1975 conference on fertility transition in Kyoto, Japan, supplemented by specially commissioned papers. The papers are made up of county-specific reviews of demographic trends in the past, analysis of socio-cultural and demographic factors associated with these trends, and a discussion of their probable future prospects. Despite differences in the tempo of fertility declines in East Asian countries, a common pattern emerges. Among younger women, fertility decline is largely attributable to later age at marriage. The practice of contraception and abortion accounts for much of the fertility reduction among older women.

161. Cleland, J. (1993). Equity, security and fertility. A reaction to Thomas. *Population Studies,* 47 (2), pp. 345-352.

The author examines recent arguments that sustained fertility decline cannot occur in circumstances of inequality, insecurity, and injustice. The empirical record suggests that none of them act as an absolute barrier to mass adoption of birth control and subsequent fertility decline. Recent trends in Bangladesh illustrate this point vividly.The author argues that one of the greatest fallacies of many fertility theories has been the assumption that there is an economic or social imperative in underdeveloped countries for couples to have many children. On the contrary, the historic norm for all societies has been an average of only about two surviving children per woman, implying an adaptation to low, not high, net fertility.

162. Cleland, J., J.F. Phillips, S. Amin, G.M. Kamal. (1993). Fertility decline in post-independence Bangladesh: evidence from recent demographic surveys. *Population Council Research Division Working Paper,* No. 54. 70 pages. Population Council, Research Division, New York, NewYork.

This study presents evidence that Bangladesh has witnessed a substantial fertility decline in the two decades since independence. In 1975 the total fertility rate was about seven births per woman. By 1988, it had fallen to about five births per woman, equivalent to a 30 percent drop. By 1990, the TFR was about 4.5. The predominant proximate determinant of the decline has been an increase in use of contraception, which rose from about 3 percent in 1971 to 40 percent in 1991. Delayed age at marriage has also had a modest impact. The analysis shows that all major socio-economic strata have modified their reproductive behaviour.

163. Cleland, J., J.F. Phillips, S. Amin, & G.M. Karmal. (1994). *The Determinants of Reproductive Change in Bangladesh. Success in a Challenging Environment.* Washington D.C. The World Bank, 1994, 187 pages.

The study looks at the recent fertility change in Bangladesh. It has three broad components. The third part of the book by far the longest, considers what the authors see as the true explanation of the fertility decline. Supply-side factors in particular the provision of services by the family planning program to cater to a latent demand for birth control that would otherwise be unexpressed. The main story here is the evolution of the governments program activities, but the well-known Matlab experiment with alternative service delivery strategies are also drawn.

164. Coale, A. (1988). Fertility and mortality in different populations with special attention to China. *Proceedings of the American Philosophical Society,* 1988, 132 (2) pp. 185-195.

Following a brief introduction to the positions within the demographic transition process of developed and less developed nations, this article analyses China's population policy from 1962 onwards following the Great leap forward. Family planning projects did not significantly reduce fertility until 1970 when policies were enforced most strongly. Due to the large numbers of births in the 1960s, a high proportion of the population is now in the childbearing range, and total fertility rates will need to be extremely low to achieve current targets. Finally the author discusses some of the economic disadvantages of low fertility, and the possibilities of applying similar techniques in other developing countries.

165. Concepcion, M.B. (1996). Population Policies and Family Planning in Southeast Asia. In W. Lutz (eds.). *The Future Population of the World. What Can We Assume Today?* Revised and Updated Edition, pp. 88-101.

This study examines the population policies and family planning programs in selected Southeast Asian countries and attempts to draw from their experience the critical preconditions for family-planning program success. The study shows that by making contraceptives easily available and by encouraging smaller families through a variety of measures, public and private sector family planning programs have heightened contraceptive use. In turn, fertility and population growth rates have been reduced.

166. Courbage, Y. (1995). Declining fertility in the Arab Peninsula. *Population* (Paris), 50 (2), pp. 415-446.

This article examines fertility differences between countries in the Arab peninsula . Factors such as delayed marriage, contraceptive use, urbanization and education might account for the vast differences between countries. The author suggests that high oil revenues might have led to more affluence and higher fertility, masking the influence of improvements in the status of women on fertility decline. The article suggests that a fall in the world price of oil might lead to fertility decline in the penninsula.

167. Das Gupta, M. (1993). Fertility decline in Punjab, India: Parallels with historical Europe. *Population Studies and Training Center Working Paper Series,* No. 93-11, Oct 1993. 22 pp. Brown University, Population Studies and Training Center, Providence, Rhode Island.

The author examines fertility decline in Punjab, India. The study also draws parallels with the European experience. It is suggested that the stability of expectations may be a key factor in initiating fertility declines.

168. Das Gupta, M. (1994). What motivates fertility decline? A case study from Punjab, India. In: *Understanding reproductive change: Kenya, Tamil Nadu, Punjab, Costa Rica,* (ed.). By B. Egero & M. Hammarskjold. 1994. 101-33 pp. Lund University Press, Lund, Sweden.

The author discusses the timing and pattern of the fertility decline and the determinants of fertility in Punjab, India, followed by an examination of the reasons underlying the onset and the acceleration of the fertility decline. The concluding section brings the findings together in a review of the applicability to the Punjab case of several of the major theories of fertility decline in the literature.

169. Degraff, D.S, R.E. Bilsborrow, & D. Guilkey. (1997). Community-level determinants of contraceptive use in the Philippines. A structural analysis. *Demography,* 34, 3, pp. 385-398.

The study uses household and community level data from the Philippines to estimate a multilevel model of contraceptive use. The results suggest that these are significant effects on fertility behaviour of community-level family planning services, labour market conditions, and infrastructure development. These results provide structural insights regarding the structural determinants of contraceptive use and fertility that are useful for drawing policy implications.

170. Dharmalingam, A. & S. P. Morgan. (1996). Women's Work, Autonomy and

Birth Control. Evidence From Two South Indian Villages. *Population Studies* Vol. 50, pp. 187-201.

The study contrasts two south Indian villages, Village I and Village II, which offer women very different employment opportunities. The study argues that greater autonomy will increase contraceptive use among women who want no more children. The study finds strong support for this hypothesis. But because there are few competing employment opportunities in Village II, women in that village have received substantially more education than those in Village I. More generally the study shows that fertility decline is occurring, and that low fertility can exist in very different settings.

171. Dissanayake L. (1996). The first generation with mass schooling and the fertility transition: the case of Sri Lanka. *Health Transition Review*, Supplement 6, pp. 137-154.

The study looks at the pre-transitional fertility regime in Sri Lanka and the factors responsible for its destabilisation.

172. Donaldson, P.J, D. J. Nicholas, H.C. Choe. (1978). Abortion and contraception in the Korean fertility transition. *Population Studies*, 36, 227.

The study examines the Korean fertility transition and looks at the influence of abortion and contraception towards the decline.

173. Dowrick, S. (1995). Demographic change, investment and growth in the Asia-Pacific region. *Asia Pacific Economic Review.* 1 (1), pp. 20-31.

Marked declines in birth rates in many Asia-Pacific countries since 1960 have caused the working-age proportion of those populations to rise substantially. The consequent increase in labour force participation is estimated to have contributed up to one percentage point increase in annual average growth rates of per capita GDP. In addition to the growth-enhancing impact of demographic transition, further econometric evidence indicates that achieving lower levels of fertility also increases the long-run per capita growth through capital deepening.

174. Duraisamy, M. (1993). Women's choice of work and fertility in urban Tamil Nadu, India. *Economic Growth Center Discussion Paper, No.* 695, June 1993.28 pp. Yale University, Economic Growth Center, New Haven, Connecticut.

The author examines the joint determinants of women's choice of work and fertility within the Nash-bargaining framework using household survey data from urban

Tamil Nadu, India. The findings of the study show that an increase in women's wage would draw more women into wage work and self-employment and concomitantly reduce fertility.

175. Dwivedi, S.N & S. Rai. (1995). Impact of some demographic variables and family planning programme on fertility in Madhya Pradesh through indirect techniques. *Health and Population Perspectives and Issues,* 18 (1), pp. 19-26.

This article investigates the impact of some demographic variables and family planning programme on fertility change. Indirect statistical tools were used for this purpose. The standardisation method was used to play with demographic variables namely age structure, marital status distribution, age specific marital fertility rate and proportion of women of reproductive ages in the total and trend analysis was used to play with family planning planning programme. It was noted that proportion of women of reproductive ages in total population played tremendous role regarding change in crude birth rate. However, there was no significant impact of family planning programme on fertility change.

176. Dyson, T. & M. Moore. (1983). On Kinship structure, female autonomy and demographic behaviour. *Population and Development Review,* 9, No 1, pp. 35-60.

The study uses a strong element of ideational or cultural factors to explain the divergence between northern and southern India. They attribute the disparity to two different sociocultural systems, which differ in both kinship system and extent of female autonomy.

177. Dyson, T. & M. Murphy. (1983). On Kinship Structure, Female Autonomy and demographic behaviour in India. *Population and Development Review,* Vol. 9, pp. 35-60.

The purpose of this article is twofold: The first is to elaborate on and confirm the relative clarity and long-term historical consistency of the dichotomous regional pattern of demographic performance. The second is to develop a sociological model of the different gender relations inherent in north south Indian culture and to describe how this model may help explain some of the differences in demographic performance.

178. Eickelman, C. (1993). Fertility and social change in Oman: women's perspectives. *Middle East Journal,* Vol. 47, No. 4, autumn, pp. 652-66.

The author examines trends in fertility and social change in Oman from an anthropological perspective. The data is based on the author's two visits in 1979 to 1980 and 1988.

179. Fawcett, J. T. & S. E. Khoo. (1980). Singapore: Rapid fertility transition in a compact society. *Population and Development Review,* 6, No 4, pp. 549-579.

The study looks at the factors underlying the rapid transition to low fertility in Singapore using a variety of sources that goes beyond the usual demographic studies. Factors contributing to this decline discussed in the paper include government policies and programs designed to influence fertility directly, policies, programs and practices in education, female employment, and public housing which influence indirectly and changing values, attitudes and aspirations of Singaporeans- particularly with respect to the value of children in the context of a society undergoing remarkable social and economic transformation.

180. Feeney, G., F. Wang., M. Zhou & B. Xiao. (1989). Recent Fertility Dynamics in China. Results from the 1987 One-percent Population Survey. *Population and Development Review,* 15, No 2, pp. 297-322.

In mid-1987 the State Statistical Bureau of China carried out a large-scale population survey titled the One-percent Population Survey. The 1-% survey canvassed a one-percent sample of China's population gathering information on some 10 million persons. This article uses data from the 1-% survey to analyse recent fertility dynamics in China. The primary objective is to learn what happened to fertility since 1982. Does the increase in crude birth rates signify a change in fertility behaviour? If so, what exactly has changed, and why? Is the long-term fertility decline that began in the 1970s intact? What are the implications, if any, for birth planning policies and programs?

181. Feeney, G. (1991). Fertility Decline in Taiwan: A study using parity progression ratios. *Demography,* 28, 3, pp. 467-479.

Taiwan's decline in fertility is studied by using period parity progression ratios. Levels of marriage and motherhood are found to have been high and essentially constant through the late 1980s, suggesting that the decline has been due almost entirely to declines in second and higher order-births. Families with three or more children play an important role in maintaining the current level of fertility. The level of fertility would be even lower without these families. They contributed more than one-half child per woman to the total fertility rate during most of the 1980s. Total fertility rates computed from the period progression ratios indicate a substantially higher level of fertility than the conventional total fertility rate; they remained above or at replacement level through 1988. A formal demographic analysis suggests that the conventional total fertility rate have been depressed by shifts in age at childbearing.

182. Feeney, G. (1994). Fertility Decline in East Asia. *Science* 266 (5190), pp.

1518-1523.

The study examines the decline in ferility in East Asia. The author argues that with the decline in fertility in China to near or below replacement levels in the early 1990s, the whole of East Asia may now be said to have completed a demographic transition. Its experience lies between that of the West and many developing countries in which demographic transition is now underway. The main features and possible causes of the fertility declines in Japan, Taiwan, South Korea, and China during this century are discussed. Fertility decline in East Asia is interesting both in its own right, as a chapter in the history of human reproduction, and for the light it may shed on fertility decline in the rest of the world.

183. Feeney, G. & Y. Jianhua (1994). Below replacement fertility in China? A close look at recent evidence. *Population Studies.* 48 (3), pp. 381-394.

This article presents detailed evidence on fertility levels and trends in China from a survey conducted in 1992 by the State Family Planning Commission. The evidence is analysed internally and by comparison with evidence from the Census of Population of 1990 and from two previous surveys. The results of the 1992 survey, which indicated fertility levels far below replacement during the early 1990s, have been greeted with considerable scepticism. Close attention has therefore been paid to evidence and argument bearing on the completeness of reporting of births in the survey. While the survey data probably understate fertility levels after 1990, the results for 1990 and before appear to be generally reliable. Even allowing for substantial underreporting of births during 1991-1992, it appears likely that Chinese fertility did, in fact, fall to replacement level during the early 1990s.

184. Feeney, G. (1996). Fertility in China. Past, Present, Prospects. In Wolfgang Lutz (eds.). *The Future Population of the World. What Can We Assume Today?* Revised and Updated Edition, pp. 102-130.

The study provides a comprehensive account of China's fertility decline at the national level, with emphasis on those factors relevant to a consideration of the future trajectory of fertility.

185. Freedman, R. (1995). Asia's recent fertility decline and prospects for future demographic change. *Asia Pacific Population Research Reports,* 1, 27 pages.

This report surveys fertility trends in Asia since the mid-1960s, focusing on 24 countries that together account for 3.1 billion, or 56 percent of the world's population. Asian fertility has declined overall by 39 percent or 62 percent of the decline necessary for reaching the population-replacement level of 2.1 children per woman, and contraceptive use has risen sharply throughout much of the region. By 1990 nine out of 10 Asians were living in countries where fertility had fallen by at least 25 percent. Although fertility rates and contraceptive use vary widely within the region, three out of four Asians today live in six countries where fertility rates range from 4.5 to 2.1 children per woman and nearly two-thirds of married couples, on average, practice contraception. The report considers three factors usually believed to account for these astonishing rapid changes in reproductive behaviour: mortality decline, broad social and economic development, and effective national family planning programs. An assessment follows of the current plausible pathways for reducing fertility, and likely future fertility levels in individual countries and sub-regions.

186. Freedman, R, M.C. Chang & T.H. Sun. (1994). Taiwan's transition from high fertility to below-replacement levels. *Studies In Family Planning,* 25, No. 6, pp. 317-331.

This article compares the fertility experience of Taiwan in the eight years since the total fertility rate reached 2.1 with that before fertility reached replacement levels. During the earlier period, two-thirds of the fertility decline resulted from falling marital fertility and one-third from higher age at marriage. The changing age distribution retarded this decline. Since 1983, the further decline to a rate of 1.7-1.8 has been entirely the result of the trend toward later marriage. Older age distributions now facilitate the decline. The question as to what would have happened without Taiwan's effective family planning program is impossible to determine, but clearly, contraceptive services supplied by the program were the major proximate cause of Taiwan's fertility decline.

187. Gertler, P & J. Molyneaux. (1994). How economic development and family planning programs combined to reduce Indonesian fertility. *Demography,* Vol. 31, No. 1, pp. 33-63.

The study examines the contribution of family planning programs, economic development and women's status to Indonesian fertility decline from 1982 to 1987. The study revealed that 75% of the fertility decline resulted from increased contraceptive use, but was induced primarily through economic development and improved education and economic opportunities for females.

188. Goldscheider, C. (ed.) (1992). *Fertility Transitions, Family Structure and Population Policy.* Brown University Studies in Population and Development Westview Press: Boulder, Colorado, Oxford, England, 283 pages.

This book focuses on fertility and fertility transitions in selected third world countries mainly drawn from Asia such as Taiwan, Indonesia, South Korea and Thailand.

189. Golstein, A. & F. Wang. (1996). China: the many facets of demographic change. *Brown University Studies in Population and Development,* 1996, 214 pp. Westview Press: Boulder, Colorado, Oxford, England.

This book is organised along eleven chapters and three themes. First, the book looks at the extent to which socio-economic changes affect demographic behaviour in China; Second, the interaction between the state and society; and finally the extent to which demographic changes will affect China's socio-economic development.

190. Gosal, G.S. (1991). Spatial patterns of fertility trends in India 1971-1987. An interpretative Study. *Kieler-Geographische-Schriften,* 78, pp. 379-388.

This study examines the dynamics of fertility change in India between the period 1971 to 1987. In terms of the spatial variations of the change the northern and southern cultural regimes stand in marked contrast to each other. This macro regional contrast has much to do with the social status and autonomy of the women as provided in their respective cultures than economic development, industrialisation and urbanisation.

191. Greenhalgh, S, Z. Chuzhu, N. Li. (1994). Restraining population growth in three Chinese villages. *Population and Development Review,* 20, (2), pp. 365-395.

The latest nation-wide survey of Chinese fertility suggests that, after rising during the mid-1980s, fertility has fallen steadily since the late 1980s, reaching replacement level in 1992. Through a restudy of three villages in the north-western province of Shaanxi, this article explores the politics and economics of this striking demographic development in a locality well known to the authors from previous research. Between 1988 and mid-1993, they find, village fertility fell to new lows due to increased emphasis on birth planning by leaders at all levels and, to a lesser extent, economic advance that reduced already very low childbearing aspirations.

192. Greenhalgh, S.; C. Zhu; N. Li, (1993). Restraining population growth in three Chinese villages: 1988-93. *Population Council Research Division Working Paper,* No, 55, 1993, 48 pages. Population Council Research Division, New York, New York.

This article describes a restudy of three villages in the northwestern province of Shaanxi (China) that were first investigated by the authors in early 1988. The earlier research explored the political economy of family and fertility change during the decades 1947-87. In mid-1993 the authors went back to the villages to discover how fertility had changed in the previous six years, and why. They found out that fertility fell to new lows due to increased emphasis on birth planning by leaders at all levels and, to a lesser extent, continued economic advance.

193. Greenspan, A. (1994). After the demographic transition: policy responses to low fertility in four Asian countries. *Asia Pacific and Policy.* 30, 4 pages.

The 1994 issue of the Asia Pacific and Policy Journal outlined the policy challenges facing Asian countries that have made the demographic transition from high to low fertility. This issue continues the discussion by surveying the fertility situation in four countries and examining their policy responses. The countries are South Korea, Taiwan, Singapore and Thailand.

194. Guest, P. & A. Chamratithirong. (1992). The Social Context Of Fertility Decline in Thailand. In Calvin Goldscheider (ed.), *Fertility Transitions, Family Structure, and Population Policy*, pp 67-99. Boulder, Col.: Westview Press.

The study uses a multilevel model to assess fertility levels and trends in Thailand. The results show that social context is a significant factor, independent of, and in addition to individual characteristics in explaining fertility decline in Thailand.

195. Guest, P. & J. Gavin. (1996). Policy options when population growth slows. The case of Thailand. *Population Research and Policy Review,* 15, 2 pp. 109-130.

Population policy in Thailand is assessed in light of rapid declines in fertility rates. Since the 1970s, that policy has sought to reduce fertility through active family planning and to distribute population away from urban Bangkok. It is argued that this trend is unlikely to reverse, and policy should focus less on fertility and more on population distribution and quality.

196. Guo, S. (1996). Determinants of fertility decline in Shanghai: development or policy? In: *China: the many facets of demographic change,* edited by Alice Goldstein and Wang Feng. 1996. 81-96 pages. Westview Press: Boulder, Colorado, Oxford, England.

This study examines the relative importance of family planning programs in urban China's fertility decline, by examining the situation in Shanghai- the largest city and, socioeconomically, the most developed area in the country. The study begins with a brief review of the trends of fertility decline in Shanghai and a discussion of the theoretical issues. Two models are then posited to depict the relative importance of the government's family planning in different periods. These findings are finally used to summarise the fundamental factors in the dramatic fertility decline in Shanghai and in urban China in general.

197. Gupta, M.D. (1995). Fertility Decline in Punjab, India: Parallels with

Historical Europe. *Population Studies,* 49, 3 pp. 481-500.

The study looks at fertility decline in 11 villages in the Ludhiana district of rural Punjab, India. It is based on historical and anthropological research as well as demographic surveys. The results of the study show that peasant families in this society traditionally used marriage regulation to keep family size in line with available land, as did their counterparts in historical Europe. It is noted that those interventions that generated a feeling of stability of expectations built up a demand for fertility control so that fertility decline began before the advent of the family planning program. It is concluded that strong parallels exist between Punjab in the 1940s and late nineteenth-century Europe, because both settings included high infant mortality rates, widespread illiteracy, and fertility decline. It is concluded that the link between development and fertility decline is the sense of stability and control over life that the former creates.

198. Gupta, M.D. & P. N. Mari Bhat. (1997). Fertility decline and increased manifestation of sex bias in India. *Population Studies,* Vol. 51, No 3, pp. 307-315.

The study explores the relations between fertility decline and the net manifestation of sex bias as well as evidence that this bias has increased in India. The study argues that the effect of fertility decline on excess mortality of girls relative to that of boys in India is influenced by two countervailing forces: the reduction in the number of higher-parity births which reduces net excess mortality, and the intensification of parity-specific discrimination which increase it. Rising sex ratios of children between 1981 and 1991 indicate that the net effect of these forces was an increase in the excess mortality of girls during this period.

199. Hirschman, C, & P. Guest. (1990). Multilevel Models of Fertility Determination in Four Southeast Asian Countries 1970 and 1980. *Demography,* vol. 27, No. 3.

The study uses micro level data from the census reports of 1970 and 1980 to test multilevel models of fertility determination for four Southeast Asian Societies.

200. Hirschman, C. & P. Guest. (1990). The Emerging demographic transitions of Southeast Asia. *Population and Development Review,* 16 No 1, pp. 121-152

Micro level data from the 1970 and 1980 censuses are used to examine fertility declines in four Southeast Asian countries: Indonesia, Malaysia, the Philippines, and Thailand. Despite the wide variations across countries, clear evidence emerges of significant fertility declines in all four countries.

201. Hirschman, C., J. Tan, A. Chamratrithirong., & P. Guest. (1993). Explaining

the rapid fertility decline in Thailand. *Seattle Population Research Center Working Paper*, No. 93-13, Aug 1993. 38 pp. University of Washington, Seattle.

The study looks at the relative role of various factors in determining the decline in fertility in Thailand during the late 1960s to the late 1970s. A multilevel model, which makes use of both structural and individual level factors, is used in the analysis. The results indicate the importance of women's status and economic roles of children in influencing the decline in fertility.

202. Hirschman, C., J. Tan., A. Chamratrithirong, & P. Guest. (1993). The path to below replacement-level fertility in Thailand. *Seattle Population Research Center Working Paper*, No. 93-12, Aug. 22 (4) pp. University of Washington, Seattle Population Research Center, Seattle, Washington, Battelle Seattle Research Center, Seattle, Washington.

Annual fertility rates for Thailand are presented for the 1980s based on data from official sources. The analysis suggests that below replacement fertility was reached by the late 1980s.

203. Hosaain, S.I. (1989). Effect of public programs on family size, child education and health. *Journal of Development Economics*, 30 (1), pp. 145-158.

The bulk of public resources in developing countries is devoted to the subvention of population control and health investments. The effects of these programs have been evaluated in this study with household and community data from Bangladesh. The results suggest that subsidy on family planning and secondary school would be most effective in the achievement of harmonious goals of reducing fertility and mortality and fostering investments in child education.

204. Hull, T.H. (1996). Continuing demographic transitions in Asia. *Asian Pacific Economic Literature*, 10 (1), pp. 42-53.

This article provides an update of the literature survey on demographic trends and policies in Asia published in the May 1987 issue of the Asian Pacific Economic Literature Journal. A report is made of substantial adjustments in earlier population projections, suggesting slower decline in population growth rates for China and several other Asian countries. It also provides an account of recent trends and policies in the Asian pacific region, especially China, Vietnam, Indonesia, the Philippines and Singapore.

205. Hunter, I.; H.B.M. Hilderink; F.J. Willekens; L.W. Niessen. (1996). Fertility Change in India. *GLOBO Report Series*, NO 13, Sept 90 pages. University of Groningen, Population Research Center. Groningen, Netherlands; Rijksinstituut Voor

Volksgezondheid en Milieu (RIUM): Bilthoven, Netherlands.

The report provides a recent discussion of fertility change in India. Some of the topics discussed include the demographic transition in India, a qualitative account of the fertility process, case studies involving the states of Uttar Pradesh and Kerela, and a description of an integrated system approach to fertility change.

206. Hutaserani, S. & J. Roumasset. (1991). Institutional change and the Demographic Transition in Rural Thailand. *Economic Development and Cultural Change*, 40 (1), pp. 75-100.

This article looks at the nature of the rural transformation and fertility decline in Thailand and to explain the relationship between the two. It begins by sketching a fertility decision-making model of farm households within the New Household Economics framework. The model incorporates primary characteristics of Thailand's rural transformation as determinants.

207. Institute of Resource Development (IRD). Declines in Fertility and Mortality slowing in Indonesia. *Demographic and Health Surveys Newsletter,* 1996, Vol. 8, No. 1.

Based on the 1994 Indonesian Demographic and Health Survey the study concludes that levels of fertility and mortality continue to decline in Indonesia but at a slower pace than before.

208. Jain, A. K & A.L. Adlakha (1982). Preliminary estimates of fertility decline in India during the 1970s. *Population and Development Review,* 8, No. 3 pp. 589-606.

The purpose of this study is two-fold: first, to provide in the interim, alternative estimates of fertility decline in India during the 1970s by using an indirect method based on the Bongaarts model (1978) of proximate determinants of fertility; and. second, to derive estimates of the fertility levels for 1972 and 1978. The findings of the study reveal that the crude birth rate in India declined by about 8 to 14 percent, from 40.6 births per 1000 population in 1972 to 35-37 in 1978, and that the decline was primarily a result of actual change in age specific fertility rates. Fertility during the 1970s is estimated to have declined in all age groups. The fertility decline in the younger age groups reflects the effect of rising age at marriage, whereas the substantial declines among women over age 25 reflect increased use of fertility control methods.

209. Jain, A.K. (1985). The impact of development and population policies on fertility in India. *Studies in Family Planning,* 16 (4), pp. 181-98.

This study looks at the role of development and population policies on fertility decline and regional variations in India during the 1970s. Indicators of development at the household level include female literacy and education, infant mortality, and poverty, at the village level they include availability of such social services as schools, medical facilities, and transportation and communication facilities. Based on a multiple regression analysis of data aggregated at the state level, the study shows that demonstrates that conditions conducive to fertility decline include high adult female literacy and low infant mortality as indicators of social development, and high contraceptive use, and to a lesser extent, high female age at marriage as proximate determinants of fertility. The study argues that there are reasons to believe that India's national family planning program contributed to the decline in fertility observed since the 1960s. The pace of fertility decline in the future will depend upon the pace of infant mortality decline, enhancement in female education, and improvements in family planning programs.

210. James, K.S. (1995). Demographic transition and education in Kerela. *Economic and Political Weekly,* Vol. 30, No. 51, pp. 3274-6.

The author examines the impact of education on fertility decline in the Indian State of Kerela against the background of the State government's decision to close 67 schools in the period 1990-1993 due to declining numbers of children of school age.

211. Jayatilake, M.J.J. (1992). *Socio-economic development and fertility decline in Sri Lanka.* PhD. dissertation Vanderbilt University. 221 pages.

The study examines the causes; timing and magnitude of the decline in fertility in Sri Lanka between 1963 to 1981 based on census data. Multiple regression analysis is used in analysing the data.

212. Jeffrey, R. & A.M. Basu. (Eds.) (1996). *Girls Schooling, Women's Autonomy and Fertility Change in South Asia.* New Delhi. Sage Publications. 339 pages.

The book originated from a 1993 workshop held in New Delhi. It questions the conventional wisdom that female education raises women's autonomy and thereby lower fertility. While fully supporting female schooling and female adult literacy campaigns, the editor's caution against any simple presumption that such measures will necessarily bring about fertility (or mortality) reductions.

213. Jejeebhoy, S.J. (1984). The Shift from natural to controlled fertility. A Cross-sectional analysis of ten Indian States. *Studies in Family Planning,* 15, (4), pp. 191-8.

The objective of the study was to assess the causes of the fertility transition from natural to controlled fertility in India by comparing couples who had used contraceptives with those who remained under natural fertility conditions. The results of the study revealed that it is primarily improvements in child mortality and its effects through intervening factors, which account for the transition.

214. Jones, G.W. (ed.) (1984). *Demographic Transition in Asia.* Singapore. Maruzen Asia. 231 pages.

This book provides a readable and authoritative account of recent demographic trends in the major countries of Asia. It addresses three demographic trends in region wide issues: the process of transition and whether it has stalled, the pace of improvement in health and life expectancy and its determinants, the changing patterns of internal migration. There often seems an underlying premise that government delivery of family planning services is necessary for fertility decline.

215. Jones, G.W. (1990). Fertility Transitions among Malay Populations of Southeast Asia: Puzzles of Interpretation. *Population and Development Review,* 16, pp. 507-537.

Fertility trends among Malay populations of Southeast Asia raise questions about alternative theories of fertility decline. Singapore Malays, urbanised and the wealthiest among the populations under review, reached replacement level fertility in 1975. Indonesians, the least urbanised and lowest income group have experienced substantial declines in fertility. The Malays of Peninsula Malaysia have had lesser fertility declines than the Indonesians, and their fertility rose over an eight-year period following 1978. All of these Malay populations have experienced rising income, albeit from widely differing base levels, expansion of education, the communications revolution, and increasing consumerism. But the political and institutional settings differed. Elements of demand theory, diffusion theory, and institutional approaches need to be invoked in explaining these fertility trends.

216. Jowett, A.J. (1989). China. *The Demographic Disaster of 1958-1961. In Population and Disaster.* Edited by J.I. Clarke, P. Curson, S. L. Kayastha and P. Nag. Blackwell, Oxford, UK, pp. 137-158.

The study looks at demographic responses to the famine in China during the late 1950s and early 1960s. Famine conditions were responsible for halving of fertility between 1957 and 1961 with the TFR declining precipitously from 6.405 to 3.287. The study notes that the demographic response to the famine appears to correspond closely with the general model postulated by Bongaarts and Cain for developing countries. A variety of mechanisms appear to link nutritional deprivation with temporary infertility: reduced libido in females and males, decrease coital frequency and reduction in the production of sperm; separation of spouses while searching for food, and famine amenorrhoea, which was widely reported in China, generated widespread temporary sterility.

217. Karra, M.V, N. N. Stark, & J. Wolf. (1997). Male Involvement in Family Planning. A Case Study Spanning Five Generations of a South Indian Family. *Studies in Family Planning,* 28, 1, pp. 24-34.

This study examines fertility decisions made by five generations of one South Indian family and the factors affecting its sudden observed fertility decline. The involvement of males in family planning and use of male methods are associated with the fertility decline and resulted in long-term benefits for women. Traditional notions about gender roles and family, in addition to economic concerns, shaped fertility decision making.

218. Khander, S.R. & M.A. Latif. (1996). The role of family planning and targeted credit programs in demographic change in Bangladesh. *World Bank Discussion Papers.* 337, 32 pages.

The study examines the extent to which family planning programs contributed to the recent fertility decline in Bangladesh, and whether alleviating poverty through credit programs for the poor could improve contraceptive use and thereby reduce fertility and infant mortality. The study notes that while these might serve to curtail both infant mortality and fertility, these are only short-term measures. It is recommended that working towards raising the education levels of both men and women would raise productivity which would in turn increase contraceptive use and reduce infant mortality and fertility.

219. Kim, D. (1992). Sociodemographic Determinants of the Fertility Transition in Korea. In Calvin Goldscheider (ed.). *Fertility Transitions, Family Structure & Population Policy,* pp. 45-65.

The author explores the theoretical basis of the Korean fertility transition and looks at the interrelations between mortality as well as migration in the process of the transition.

220. Kim, I. (1996). Demographic Transition and Population Ageing in Korea. *Korea Journal of Population and Development,* 25, 1.

The study examines the process of population ageing in conjunction with the demographic transition in South Korea, where rapid decreases of both the mortality and fertility rates have brought about the process of population ageing.

221. Kishor, S. (1994). Fertility decline in Tamil Nadu, India. In *Understanding*

reproductive change: Kenya, Tamil Nadu, Punjab, Costa Rica, (ed.). B. Egero and M. Hammarskjold. 1994, pp. 65-100. Lund University Press, Lund, Sweden.

This study provides an evaluation of the pace and timing of decline in fertility in Tamil Nadu (India) and to identify the socio-economic, cultural, and institutional factors responsible for it. The study first traces the trends in fertility and other relevant demographic variables in Tamil Nadu, concentrating on the period 1970-1990. Then it discusses Tamil Nadu's recent socio-political history, and compares Tamil Nadu's economic and social development in the post-independence period, to that of other major Indian states. Finally, it examines the role of the official family planning program in promoting contraception in Tamil Nadu.

222. Knodel, J, N. Havanon, W. Sittitrai. (1990). Family Size and the education of children in the context of rapid fertility decline. *Population and Development Review,* 16 (1), pp. 31-62.

Results of a survey of semi-matched samples in two rural sites in Thailand indicate that family size has an important impact on children's education. The number of children in a family and the likelihood that a child will study beyond the compulsory level are inversely associated, even when other important determinants of children's schooling are controlled. Survey results and qualitative data collected through focus groups also reveal that in Thailand the primary responsibility for funding children's education falls directly on parents. Thus, more children readily translate into reduced resources available per child and hence less education. Given the inverse association between family size and children's education, the fertility decline that is under way is likely to contribute to rising levels of education by changing the distribution of children with respect to family size.

223. Knodel, J, N. Chayovan, S. Siriboon. (1992). The impact of fertility decline on familial support for the elderly. An illustration from Thailand. *Population and Development Review.* 18, (1), pp. 79-103.

The recent reduction in the number of children among Thai couples is perceived as one of the most important social changes likely to affect the support of the elderly. This study suggests that the impact of fertility on familial support for the elderly may not necessarily be a key issue in decisions on whether to implement fertility reduction policies.

224. Knodel, J, N. Havanon & A. Pramualratana. (1984). Fertility Transition in Thailand. A qualitative analysis. *Population and Development Review,* 12, 2, pp. 297-325.

The study provides a qualitative analysis of the fertility transition in Thailand based on data from focus group sessions with men and women who built their families before the Thai fertility decline and with a younger generation whose members are limiting family size to two or three children. Certain components of the fertility transition are identified. First, the changes in social and economic change, causing couples to view large numbers of children as a burden. Second, a cultural setting conducive to acceptance of fertility control, and third, the availability of effective means of fertility regulation through the natural family planning programmes.

225. Knodel J, A. Chamratrithirong, N. Debavalya. (1987). *Thailand's Reproductive Revolution: Rapid Fertility Decline in a Third World Setting*, Madison: University of Wisconsin Press.

Thailand's rapid fertility decline is assessed. The study shows the importance of the quantity-quality trade off, whereby families begin to have fewer children so as to invest in more schooling for each other.

226. Koening, M.A, J.F. Phillips, R.S. Simmons, M.A. Khan. (1987). Trends in family size preferences and contraceptive use in Matlab, Bangladesh. *Studies in Family Planning*, 18, (3), pp. 117-27.

The Matlab Family Planning and Health Services Project has in its ten years of existence recorded a remarkable rise in contraceptive use and a corresponding decline in fertility. This study examines the relationship between prevailing family size preferences and contraceptive use in the Matlab area between 1977 and 1984. The main factor accounting for increased contraceptive use appears to be the sharp rise in the use of contraception for the spacing of births. There also appears to be a modest increase in the percentage of women wanting no more children. These and other findings are evaluated in the light of their implications for the ongoing debate on the contribution of family planning programs to fertility decline in developing countries.

227. Kumaran, T.V. & S. A. Norbert. (1989). Family welfare planning programmes in Tamil Nadu. An appraisal of fertility trends. *Geographia medica*, 19, pp. 35-54.

This article examines family welfare planning programmes on fertility trends in Tamil Nadu. The focus however is on fertility decline. The decline is assessed in terms of crude birth rates, standardised birth rates adjusted for age structure of females 15-49 years of age and standardised birth rates adjusted for both age structure and marital status. The study argues that in order to fully understand the manner in which fertility has declined over the period of time, it is important one looks at fertility in the period before the active introduction and functioning of an intensive programme as well as during such a programme so that the relative trend analysis shows the family welfare planning programmes effects on fertility.

228. Ladier-Fouladi, M. (1996). The fertility transition in Iran. *Population* (Paris). 51, 6, pp. 1101-1127.

Iran experienced a significant fertility decline during the second half of the 1980s after a long persistent high fertility. A close examination of both close and remote determinants clearly shows that evolving sociocultural and economic circumstances are the principal cause of fertility decline.

229. Lavely, W.R. (1986). Age patterns of Chinese marital Fertility, 1950-1981. *Demography,* Vol. 23, No 3, pp. 419-434.

This article examines Chinese marital fertility in rural and urban sectors and finds unusual and distinctive patterns of transition from uncontrolled to controlled fertility.

230. Leete, R. (1991). Fertility trends and prospects in east and Southeast Asian countries and implications for policies and programmes. *Population Research Leads,* No. 39, 1991. 17 pages. United Nations Economic and Social Commission for Asia and the Pacific.

The author provides a comparative examination of fertility patterns and projections in selected countries in eastern and south eastern Asia as well as their political and socio-economic changes. Some of the items covered include marriage patterns; female labour force participation and it effect on fertility, and social policy development. A discussion of population policies, family planning programmes and contraception and their roles in the fertility transition in Asia is also made.

231. Leete, R. & I. Alan. (1993). (Eds.). *The Revolution in Asian Fertility. Dimensions Causes and Implications.* Oxford. Clarendon Press, 1993, 329 pages.

This study consists of a collection of articles on Asian fertility decline that emerged from an IUSSP meeting. Cases of dramatic fertility declines are found both at the national and sub-national levels. Among countries, China, the two Koreas, Taiwan, Thailand, Singapore, Hong Kong and Sri Lanka have experienced the largest falls, their fertility now half their peak levels or less. Among states or provinces elsewhere, a longer list would start with Kerela, Tamil Nadu, East Java and Bali.

232. Leete, R. (1996). *Malaysia's demographic transition: rapid development, culture, and politics.* 1996, 222 pages. Oxford University Press: Kuala Lumpur, Malaysia.

The study provides a record of demographic changes that have occurred in Malaysia since 1957. The emphasis is on changes and differentials in fertility behaviour, their causes and their consequences. Topics discussed include the dimensions of the fertility changes that have occurred, at differing paces and to differing degrees, among the three major communities in the states of Peninsular Malaysia since independence in 1957. Accounts of demographic changes that have occurred among the main communities in the lesser-developed states of Sabah and Sarawak since 1960 are also discussed. The likely demographic scenario that Malaysia will follow as it progresses towards becoming a fully developed nation targeted for the year 2020 is finally given.

233. Lee-Jay, C. & L.G. Martin. (1990). Foreign investment and demographic dynamics of the Asia-Pacific region. *Asian Economic Journal,* 4 (1), pp. 46-68.

The study looks at the role of foreign investment on demographic dynamics of the Asia-Pacific region. It argues that in recent years, the Asia-Pacific region has received world wide recognition for its remarkable economic growth. Perhaps less widely recognised by economists is the extraordinary success of many of the regions countries over the same period in reducing birth, death and population growth rates. The pace of demographic transition from high fertility and mortality to low fertility and mortality in the Asia-Pacific region has been much faster than that experienced historically in the west and currently in Latin America and Africa. The study argues that these two phenomena of rapid economic development and demographic transition are linked not only by interactions that are internal to each country, but also by the effects of neighbouring countries economic and demographic changes.

234. Le Grand, T.K & J.F. Phillips. (1996). The Effect of fertility reductions on infant and child mortality. Evidence from Matlab in Rural Bangladesh. *Population Studies,* 50, pp. 51-68.

This article uses data from Matlab, Bangladesh to assess the net effect of falling total fertility on mortality rates of young children. Real time-series models are estimated to determine the role of fertility decline after having controlled for the effects of other health service interventions. The findings of the study reveal that fertility reductions have little effect on neonatal and postneonatal mortality, possibly a small effect on toddler (second year) mortality, and a significant and relatively large impact on the mortality of children aged between 2 and 4 years. Possible explanations for these findings and their implication are discussed.

235. Li, W. & Z. Liang. (1993). The change of fertility patterns in rural and urban China, 1970-1989. *China Population Today,* Vol. 10, No.5, pp. 13-5. Beijing, China.

An analysis of fertility change in rural and urban areas of China is made based on data from Two Per Thousand Survey on Fertility and Contraception in 1988 and the 1990 population census. The Total Fertility Rate (TFR) showed a declining trend in the last two decades, though a difference still remains in the fertility level between rural and urban areas. The significant decrease of the total fertility rate for the third and higher parity births is the major cause for the rapid decline in TFR. Changes in age at first birth for urban and rural women are also considered, as well as changes in age at higher-parity births.

236. Li, W.L. (1973). Temporal and spatial analysis of Fertility Decline in Taiwan. *Population Studies,* pp. 97-104.

This article looks at the spatial and temporal dimensions of fertility decline in Taiwan. The study first presents the temporal development of fertility changes in terms of their possible relation with declining mortality and increasing educational level. It then evaluates the impact of family planning programmes on fertility decline. And third, it assesses whether such institutional variables as mortality decline and educational level influenced fertility. The findings generally substantiate the hypotheses, but with certain qualifications. For instance the relation varies according to community characteristics, the effect of infant mortality appears to be more important in rural townships, but the educational effect in cities is more discernible.

237. Limanonda, B. (1992). Nuptiality Patterns in Thailand: Their Implications for Further Fertility Decline. In Calvin Goldscheider (ed.), *Fertility Transitions, and Family Structure and Population Policy,* pp. 101-120.

The author examines the role of nuptiality change in Thailand as well as the potential contribution of nuptiality changes to the continuing Thai fertility transition. The study revealed that the decline was associated with strong and comprehensive family planning program initiated by the government, which has contributed to the increased use of contraception among Thai couples. In contrast, the increase in proportion single and the postponement of marriage has contributed only modestly to the reduction of fertility.

238. Lund, R. (1993). Gender Locality, and Changing Resource Management Practices. The Dry Zone of Sri Lanka. *Gender Studies Occasional Paper 5.* Gender and Development Studies Unit Asian Institute of Technology Bangkok.

The author argues that the shortage of land in the dry zone of Sri Lanka has led to a reconceptualisation of children as a resource. The ideal number of children is declining in response to the constantly diminishing access to land. Thus there is a realisation that having a large number of children may often be more of a problem than a resource.

239. Mahadevan, K. & M. Sumangala. (1987). *Social Development, Cultural Change and Fertility Decline. A Study of Fertility Change in Kerela.* New Delhi.

Sage Publications, 190 pages.

Kerela is often cited as an example of a population experiencing fertility and mortality decline in the absence of significant economic development. This book presents the findings of an in-depth study of one village in Kerela and one in Andhra Pradesh (also in South India). The methodology includes both sample surveys through an open-ended questionnaire for interviewing women and men, and case studies of selected individuals and institutions. The authors findings of the diminishing value of a second son in Kerela because of the increasing likelihood of the first sons survival is indicative of further demographic transition in that state.

240. McNicoll, G. (1982). Recent Demographic Trends in Indonesia. *Population and Development Review*, 8, No 4, pp. 811-819.

Indonesia's population trends in the 1970s are described on the basis of findings from the 1980 census. Mortality has steadily improved, although it remains high by regional standards. The TFR fell by 17 percent over the decade to the late 1970s with Java and Sumatra showing the largest declines. Projections assuming a substantial slowing of the growth rate still indicate a population of 200 million by the year 2000.

241. McNicoll, G. (1993). Strategies of fertility control: strong persuasion. *Working Papers in Demography*, Australian National University, Research School of Social Sciences, Canberra, Australia. No. 41, 1993. 16 pages.

The author explores the ethics of measures designed to put social, administrative, or economic pressure on individuals in order to bring down fertility using examples from China, India, and Indonesia.

242. Mita, R. & R. S. Simmons. (1995). Diffusion of the culture of contraception: Program Effects on Young Women in Rural Bangladesh. *Studies in Family Planning*, Vol. 26, No 1. pp. 1-13.

The study describes a process of diffusion of family planning information, ideas and technology among an unanticipated audience of young, unmarried women in rural Bangladesh. The study suggests that the Matlab family planning worker acted as a catalyst in the diffusion of new ideas and information about family planning to young, unmarried women who were not targeted by formal program strategies.

243. Montgomery, M.R & J.B. Casterline. (1993). The Diffusion of Fertility Control in Taiwan. Evidence from Pooled Cross-Section Time Series Models. *Population Studies,* 47, pp. 457-479.

The study uses areal level data to examine the possible effects of diffusion in accounting for fertility control in Taiwan. The study sees no need in tying the concept of diffusion to changes in the costs of fertility control. They argue that it can as easily accommodate changes in the perceived benefits of control.

244. Morgan, S. P. & B. B. Niraula. (1995). Gender, Inequality and Fertility in Two Nepali Villages. *Population and Development Review,* 2, No, 3 pp. 541-561.

The study uses data from two Nepali villages to advance our understanding of the relationship between gender inequality and fertility. The thesis is that greater female autonomy reduces fertility. The findings of the study support this claim as differences in women's autonomy are important determinants of fertility differences in the two villages.

245. Nag, M. & N. Kak. (1984). Demographic transition in a Punjab Village. *Population and Development Review,* No 4, pp. 661-678.

In 1970 a study by Mahmood Mamdani in Punjab concluded that there was no evidence that family planning programs were having any impact in the village. A follow up study in 1982 revealed an increase in contraceptive practice and a decline in desired family size among all caste groups in the village. The economic value of children seems to have declined significantly.

246. Nguyen, V. P., J. Knodel, M. Van Cam, & H. Xuyen. (1996). Fertility and Family Planning in Vietnam: Evidence from the 1994 Inter-Censal Demographic Survey. *Studies in Family Planning*, 27 (1), pp. 1-17.

The 1994 inter-censal Demographic Survey held in Vietnam reveals a substantial change in recent years in reproductive behaviour and attitudes. There has been a continuous decline in fertility levels, contraceptive knowledge has broadened and family size preferences have experienced a noticeable downward shift. All these suggest that Vietnam is undergoing a fertility transition which is likely to lead to low levels of fertility in the near future.

247. Niraula, B. B.; Morgan, S.P. (1995). Son and daughter preferences in Benighat, Nepal: Implications for fertility transition. *Social Biology,* 42. (3-4), pp. 256-273.

The study looks at the influence of sex preference on fertility decline in Nepal based on data from Benighat.

248. Ogino, M. (1993). Japanese women and the decline of the birth rate. *Reproductive Health Matters,* No 1. May 78-84 pages. London.

Possible causes and implications of the declining birth rate in Japan are discussed, with a focus on historical trends, policy changes, and women's reactions. The study also examines the role of economic factors and of women's growing unwillingness to bear the burden of child rearing is considered.

249. Paydarfar, A. A. & R. Moini. (1995). Modernisation process and fertility change in pre-and post-Islamic revolution of Iran: a cross-provincial analysis, 1966-1986. *Population Research and Policy Review*. (14), pp. 71-90.

The purpose of this article is to examine some of the possible causal links between modernisation forces and fertility patterns of the Iranian provinces during three time periods, 1966, 1976 and 1986. A modernisation scale was constructed using Iranian census data. Six indicators of industrialisation, urbanisation and universal education were used to develop the scale. The ratio of children under 5 years per woman 15 to 44 years old was used as a measure of fertility. The findings show that modernisation has proceeded upward in an almost consistent pattern in all the provinces during 1966-1986.

250. Peterson, K.D. (1991). *The economics and demographies of fertility transitions: calculation or imitation*? Ph.D. Dissertation State University of New York at Stony Brook. 204 pages.

The factors affecting the decline of fertility in Sri Lanka are examined using World Fertility Survey and Demographic and Health Survey data.

251. Phai, N. V; J. Knodel; M. Van Cam; H. Xuyen. (1996). Fertility and Family Planning in Vietnam: Evidence from the 1994 Inter-censal Demographic Survey. *Studies in Family Planning*, Vol. 27, No 1, pp. 1-17.

The findings of the study suggest that Vietnam is in the midst of a transition that will lead to low levels of fertility in the near future.

252. Phillips, J. F; R. S. Simmons, M.A. Koening, and J. Chakraborty. (1988). Determinants of reproductive change in a traditional society. Evidence from Matlab, Bangladesh. *Studies in Family Planning*, 19 (6 pt 1), pp. 313-34.

It is more than a decade since the Matlab project was launched in Bangladesh to test the hypothesis that contraceptive services can induce and sustain fertility decline in a rural traditional population. The demographic impact of this project has been pronounced, lending support to the view that supply-side policies can succeed where institutional supports for demand are weak. This article reviews the relationship between the Bangladesh climate of demand and the Matlab stayem of supply with the aim of explaining how such effects arise. A sociologically appropriate system of supply can induce fertility change in a society where such change would not spontaneously arise. The study of programs and the sociology of the supply side thus deserve the same degree of rigor accorded research on the sociology of demand.

253. Pong, S. (1994). Sex preference and fertility in Peninsular Malaysia. *Studies in Family Planning,* Vol. 25, No.3, May-June 1994. 137-48 pp. New York , New York.

Data from the Second Malaysian Family Life Survey, conducted in 1988 is used to examine parent's preferences for the sex of their children within each of Malaysia's three ethnic groups. The findings of the study reveal that while Malay and Indian parents do not show a consistent sex preference. Chinese parents prefer to have all sons, or a combination of sons and daughters, with more sons than daughters, or at least an equal number of them. The study also reveals that son preference among the Chinese does not seem to be a constraint to fertility decline among that population. Since 1970, Chinese fertility has dropped rapidly, at the same time, Chinese son preference has become more pronounced. It is further argued that further reductions in Chinese fertility, through the reduction in sex preference, would be small.

254. Raftery, A.E; S. Lewis & A. Aghajanian. (1995). Demand or Ideation? Evidence from the Iranian Fertility Decline. *Demography,* Vol. 32 No 2, May, pp. 159-182.

This article examines the determinants of the Iranian fertility decline and argue that structural socio-economic factors offer a major explanation for the decline rather than ideational change.

255. Ratcliffe, J. (1978). Social Justice and the Demographic Transition. Lessons from India's Kerala State. *International Journal of Health Services,* Vol. 8, No 1, pp. 123-142.

The study looks at the demographic transition in the Indian State of Kerela and offers some possible explanations. It argues that the anomalous and unexpected demographic trends and levels are not the result of the direct intervention designed to influence health and fertility levels, but rather reflect a broad social response to structural reforms in its political economy.

256. Ross, J.L.; Blangero, J.; Goldstein, M.C.; Schuler, S. (1986). Proximate determinants of fertility in the Kathmandu Valley, Nepal: An anthropological case study. *Journal of Biosocial Science,* 18 (2), pp. 179-196.

This article employs the analytical model of Bongaarts and Potter to compare the proximate determinants of fertility among three populations in Nepal's Kathmandu

Valley with the following characteristics: (1) high and low caste, (2) urban and urban fringe residence, and (3) users and non-users of contraception. It is shown that while Nepal, as a whole, is firmly entrenched in phase 1 of the fertility transition, each of the populations studied has begun to experience a demographic transition to different degrees. In fact, greater progress in controlling fertility has been made than previously known.

257. Salaff, J.W. (1985). Family size intentions and socio-economic status in Singapore, 1974-1981. *Studies in Family Planning,* 16, (4), pp. 199-210.

Singapore has in recent years experianced an extensive fertility decline which has affected couples at all socioeconomic levels. This article compares child bearing intentions with actual child bearing behaviour among 45 young Chinese Singaporean couples. The couples; ranked as average, affluent working class or middle class; were first interviewed in 1974-76 and followed up in 1981. The study found that on average, all the couples in the sample bore 0.4 fewer children than originally intended, though the reasons for the change differed according to socioeconomic status and the perceived role of children in the family economy.

258. Sathar, Z.A. (1993). The much-awaited fertility decline in Pakistan: wishful thinking or reality? *International Family Planning Perspectives,* Vol. 19, No.4, Dec 1993, pp 142-6. New York, New York.

The study uses demographic data from Pakistan covering the past 30 years to examine whether the country is experiencing the beginning of a fertility transition. Emphasis is given to total fertility rates, trends in proximate variables, including marriage, age and breast-feeding prevalence, and supply and demand factors affecting fertility, including child-rearing costs and child value. An analysis of Pakistan's family planning policies and programs is also made.

259. Sathar, Z.A & K.O. Mason. (1993). How female education affects reproductive behaviour in urban Pakistan. *Asian and Pacific Population Forum,* 6 (4) pp. 93-103.

This article explores the routes through which female education affects fertility in urban Pakistan. It first considers whether the inverse association between female education and cumulative fertility can be explained entirely by such variables as marriage duration and the extent of breastfeeding, known as child supply variables. Having found that supply factors do not explain the relationship completely, it considers demand factors and fertility-regulation costs as possible explanations. The results suggest that a combination of supply, demand and fertility regulation factors explains the negative relationship between education and fertility, implying that increased investment in education for females could encourage significant fertility decline in urban Pakistan.

260. Savitri, R. (1994). Fertility rate decline in Tamil Nadu: some issues. *Economic and Political Weekly*, Vol. 29, no. 29, Jul 16, pp. 1850-2. Bombay, India.

The study looks at how Indian state of Tamil Nadu has been able to achieve a reduction in fertility without creating the preconditions generally associated with such a decline, such as reduced infant mortality, improved rates of literacy, and improvements in women's status. The study concludes that availability of better roads, which facilitate contact between rural and urban areas, is one of the two major factors associated with lower fertility. The other is child mortality.

261. Saw, S.H. (1990). Ethnic fertility differentials in Peninsular Malaysia and Singapore. *Journal of Biosocial Science*, 22, (1), pp. 101-12.

Differences in fertility between the three major ethnic groups (Malays, Chinese and Indians) in Peninsular Malaysia and Singapore have existed since before the onset of fertility decline in the late 1950s and remain today, although the relative positions and the actual differences have changed due to the varying rates of decline. By 1987, the Malays experienced the highest fertility and the Chinese the lowest in both countries but in Singapore the Malay fertility was lower than the Chinese fertility in Peninsular Malaysia. The study concludes that the fertility differentials will lead to changes in the ethnic composition in both countries but more so in Peninsular Malaysia.

262. Schuler, S., S.M. Hashemi, A.P. Riley. (1997). The influence of women's changing roles and status in Bangladesh's fertility transition: evidence from a study of credit programs and contraceptive use. *World Development*, Vol. 25, No 4, pp. 563-75.

Multivariate analyses of data from a previous study in rural Bangladesh suggest that women's access to credit provided by two organisations, Grameen Bank and BRAC, augments use of contraception. The authors present qualitative data describing how the credit programs empower women and speculate about other paths through which participation in them may influence contraceptive use.

263. Shah, I.H.; T.W. Pullum; M. Irfan. (1986). Fertility in Pakistan during the 1970s. *Journal of Biosocial Science*, 18 (2), pp. 215-230.

A survey conducted in 1975, as part of the World Fertility Survey programme, provided evidence that fertility began to decline in Pakistan during the early 1970s. Because of the low level of contraceptive use recorded in that survey, the fertility decline was attributed to delayed marriage. However, a second and similar survey conducted approximately 5 years later showed almost exactly the same pattern of very recent fertility decline, and indeed a reduction in contraceptive use. The two surveys disagreed for the period of overlap. It is concluded that there were essentially no changes in fertility during the decade, and that it remained at pre-1970 levels.

264. Sharma, S, D.S. Singhal, B.B.L. Sharma, Y.P. Gupta. (1991). Factors associated with fertility moderation in India. *Asian Journal of Economic and Social Studies,* Vol. 10, No.2, Apr 1991. 137-55 pp. Muzaffarnagar, India.

Intermediate variables associated with fertility decline in India from the 1960s to 1988 are analysed based on official data sources. The emphasis is on comparisons among states as revealed primarily by data on couples protected from unwanted pregnancies by family planning methods. Among the variables used in the analysis are female age at marriage, female literacy, infant mortality, poverty, expenditure on health and family welfare, and income.

265. Simmons, R. S. (1996). Women's lives in Transition. A Qualitative Analysis of the Fertility Decline in Bangladesh. *Studies in Family Planning,* Vol. 27, No. 5, pp. 251-268.

The study utilises qualitative data derived from 21 focus group sessions with rural women to assess the transition to low fertility in Bangladesh. The findings lend support to both economic and social change as well as strong family planning program in bringing about the decline in fertility.

266. Soon, L. (1992). Determinants of fertility in Malaysia-how much do we know? *Journal of Southeast Asian Studies,* Vol. 23, No.1 Mar 1992, pp.112-32. Singapore.

The objective of this article is to review results of literature studies done on Malaysian fertility and to bring together the scattered evidence and attempt to draw inferences that will throw light on recent trends.

267. Song, R. (1993). Characteristics and causes of the fertility transition in China. *Chinese Journal of Population Science,* Vol.5, No.2, pp. 149-58. New York, New York.

The study examines the characteristics and causes of the Chinese fertility transition and draws comparisons with the European experience.

268. Sudan, F.K. (1992). *Demographic transition in South Asia.* Anmol Publications, New Delhi, India. 300 pages.

The study examines the demographic transition in South Asia. An attempt is made to analyse the facts and features of South Asian population and the demographic factors affecting the pace and level of economic and social development in the region. It is stressed that in the present context what is needed is the increase in productive capacity to support a large population on the one hand and the reduction of fertility rates on the other hand.

269. Sun, T. H. & M. C. Chang. (1992). Demographic transition and fertility control policies in Taiwan. In *Readings in population research: policy, methods and perspectives*, (Eds.). by P. Krishnan, Chi-Hsien Tuan, and Kuttan Mahadevan. 1992. 25-57. B.R. Publishing, Delhi, India.

The author's provide an analysis of the demographic transition in Taiwan and the role the family planning programme played in the process of this transition. A discussion of the prospects of future policies is also presented. It concludes that the experience in Taiwan would be useful to other developing countries in lowering their fertility-level.

270. Surbakti, S. (1983). *The link of socio-economic factors, community development and fertility behaviour.* The case of Indonesia. Ph.D dissertation Cornell University 1983. 278 pages.

The objective of the study are to identify the determinants of fertility behaviour, to develop a fertility model for Indonesia, to examine the relationship between fertility and socio-economic and environmental variables to highlight factors influencing provincial differences in fertility behaviour. The study results imply that improved family planning services and continuing intensification of contraceptive propaganda are possible strategies for reducing fertility. The government development program might also concentrate on improving education level and providing more employment.

271. Thangkasemvathana, B. (1990). *Fertility Change And Economic Development In Taiwan* (CHINA). Ph.D. Dissertation University of Missouri-Colombia. 169 Pages.

The author examined a conceptual framework of fertility change during the process of economic development using the concept of household production. The findings lend support to the following hypotheses: that fertility decreases with household capital formation, household's members, educational level and mortality rate, but increases as household income increases.

272. Thomas, N. (1993). Economic, security, culture and fertility. A reply to Cleland. *Population Studies,* 47-(2) pp. 353-359.

The author argues that Cleland's rejection of the importance of economic security to fertility gives insufficient attention to the components of Cain's theory. Cleland's superficial regard for the full meaning of insurance, and almost total neglect of the environment of risk, he argues, leads to misinterpretation of economic and demographic data. Historical trends in fertility and security in Taiwan and South Korea fail to support Cleland's view. Likewise recent fertility decline in Bangladesh is easily accommodated within the economic security fertility theory. Cleland's use of data on fertility differentials by occupation in Bangladesh is criticised on both statistical and theoretical grounds. The innovation and diffusion of family planning as an explanation of fertility decline is seen as entirely inadequate. Instead, as in the theories of Caldwell and Cain, economic processes must be understood in cultural contexts, which reflect the complexity of the real world.

273. Thomas, N. & N. Price. (1996). The Evolution of Population Policy in Rural China. *Health Policy and Planning,* 11, 1 pp. 21-29.

The one-child family policy in the People's Republic of China brought a rapid drop in fertility during the 1970s. It was eventually abandoned because the decollectivization of agriculture weakened collective institutions, undermining birth planning administration and family planning services. However, fertility declined again, however, in 1992. Reasons for this are examined, including a falling demand for children, the provision of more accessible family planning services, and restrictive population policies. The formulation and implementation of birth control policies in rural areas are discussed, and it is noted that effective implementation of local birth plans has relied on co-operation between birth planning officials and other local government officials who regulate access to resources such as land and credit without which the aspirations of ordinary people cannot be realised.

274. Uddin, M.M. (1994). Recent fertility decline in Bangladesh. In S. Kono and Yasuko (Eds.). *Fertility in Developing Countries. A Comparative study of the Demographic and Health Surveys.* IDE Statistical Data Series. No 66. Institute of Developing Economics, Tokyo, Japan, pp. 152-180.

This article examines fertility levels and trends in Bangladesh during the past two decades based on secondary data sources. The results of the study show that the government program in Bangladesh is successful. The relative decline in fertility is certainly the credit of the family planning program but the question is how far the fertility will decline in the absence of socio-economic development. Poverty, periodic disasters and traditional pronatalist values were not enough to keep fertility desires high or repulse the concerted efforts of family planning program.

275. Vosti, S.A., & M. Lipton. (1992). Population change in the wake of agricultural improvement: lessons for Pakistan. *Pakistan Development Review,* Vol. 31. No 4. Pt. 2 winter 1992, pp. 715-28. Islamabad, Pakistan.

This paper examines the impact of several types of modern agricultural technologies (developed) since the early 1960s on fertility-based demographic transitions between 1971 and 1981 at the District level in rural India. The study begins with an estimation of total fertility rates in Section II, followed by brief District-level characteristics of agriculture in Section III. Finally the results of the empirical estimation is presented in Section IV.

276. Wang, F. (1996). A decade of the one-child policy. Achievement and implications. In *China. The many faces of Demographic Change.* (Eds.). Alice Goldstein and Wang Feng. Boulder, CO. Westview Press, Chapter 6.

The author explains the important role of mortality decline in bringing China to the two-child preferred level and the traditional kinship level in making further decline difficult.

277. Westley, S.B. (1995). New survey finds fertility decline in India. *Asia Pacific Population and Policy.* 32, 4 pages.

Survey results available from the National Family Survey (NFHS), one of the most complete of its kind ever conducted in India with nearly 90,000 responses from women provide convincing evidence that fertility has declined throughout the country. There are striking differences among regions and individual states. This issue presents new information from the survey on fertility trends and family planning practices in India. The discussion focuses on the 17 most populous states plus Delhi.

278. Wirakartakusmah, M.D. (1993). Demographic transitions in Indonesia and its implications in the 21st century. In *International Population Conference Montreal 1993,* Volume 2. 1993. 259-76 pp. International Union for the Scientific Study of Population (IUSSP), Liege, Belgium.

The study provides a review of findings from the 1990 Indonesian census and from Population projections made by the University of Indonesia's Demographic Institute, with a focus on recent demographic changes and implications for the next century. Topics discussed include fertility and mortality changes, the size of the elderly population, demands for urban employment, improvements in education, illness at older ages, and women in the labour force.

279. Yang, S. & H. Zhu. (1993). China's ethnic groups: fertility change in five autonomous regions. *China Population Today,* Vol. 10, No.4, Aug 1993.8-14 pp. Beijing, China.

The study provides a comparative analysis of fertility rates among five ethnic groups living in five autonomous regions in China. The data is drawn from the 1988 fertility survey and the 1990 census. These data sources are used to estimate trends in fertility during the period 1970-1989. A significant decrease is noted among all groups, though fertility rates among these ethnic groups are still higher than those of Han nationality. Some sociocultural determinants of fertility are discussed, including marriage and age at first birth.

280. Zafar, M; N. Ford; A. Ankomah. (1995). Significance of beliefs and values in predicting fertility and contraceptive behaviour in Pakistan. *Journal of Biosocial Science,* 27, pp. 301-318.

The study sought to examine reproductive behaviour and the extent to which socio-economic and cultural and attitudinal factors affect fertility decision-making process among women in Pakistan. The results revealed that the cultural setting and tradition exert an important influence on reproductive behaviour independent of economic development.

281. Zhou, L. (1991). *Chinese Fertility Decline in Relation to Social And Economic Development,* 1949-1982. Ph.D Dissertation University Of Cincinnati, 1991, 214 Pages.

The study examines the relationship between fertility decline and socio-economic development based on data from China. The findings suggest that the decline in fertility is associated with socio-economic development as well as family planning activities. The decline of Chinese fertility, the author concludes cannot be regarded purely as an outcome of successful family planning programs.

282. Zhu, F. (1991). *The effects of family planning policy and socio-economic development on fertility decline in China 1945-1985.* M.A. Thesis Eastern Michigan University 1991, 64 pages.

Time series analysis of the relationship between socio-economic development, family planning, and fertility transition in China is analysed between 1945 to 1985. Two areas, Shanghai, a developed area and Shaanxi, an underdeveloped area, were used to examine the variability in the fertility patterns of China's sub regions due to the considerable variation in socio-economic development. The findings of the study show that socio-economic development is the underlying variable for fertility decline in the developed urban area like Shanghai. In the under developed region of Shaanxi it was found that the forced government family planning policy was the main factor related to fertility decline.

4

Fertility Decline in Sub-Saharan Africa

283. Adamchak, D.J., & M. Mbizvo. (1990). The relationship between fertility and contraceptive prevalence in Zimbabwe. *International Family Planning Perspectives,* 16, (3) pp 103-106.

The relationship between fertility and contraceptive prevalence is analysed based on data from Zimbabwe. The findings of the study lends credence to the fact that an increase in a country's contraceptive prevalence rate over time is not always consistent with the observed fertility reduction. A number of factors are given to explain this point such as irregularity of use, overlap of contraceptive use with postpartum amenorrhoea, age at marriage, and use of abortion.

284. Adamchak, D.J. & M. Mbizvo. (1993). Structural and attitudinal change: fertility decline in Zimbabwe. *Genus,* Vol. 49, no 3-4, pp. 101-13.

This study looked at the relationship of wives and husband's education, gender equality, and place of residence with children ever born in Zimbabwe based on data from the 1988 Zimbabwe Male Fertility Survey. The results of the study show that the three residence types (rural, urban high density, and urban middle class) reveal significant differences on selected variables. The multivariate analysis showed that the education of the wife was a significant negative indicator of children ever born for the younger cohort, while for the older cohort, the urban middle class residence, gender equality and husband's education were negative and significant predictors of children ever born.

285. Adamchak, D & M. Mbizvo. (1994). The Impact of Husbands' and wives' education and occupation on family size in Zimbabwe. *Journal Of Biosocial Science* Oct 26 (4), pp. 553-8

The study examines the impact of husbands' and wives' education and occupation on family size in Zimbabwe based on the results of the 1988 Male Fertility Survey. It reveals that husbands' education had a strong negative effect, and wives' education had a moderate negative effect on the number of children ever born. Contrary to the literature, wives who were not employed had significantly fewer children than those who work in agriculture, and fewer, but not significantly, than those in non-agricultural occupations.

286. Agyei-Mensah, S. (1996). New Perspective on the Fertility Situation in Sub-Saharan Africa. *Norsk Geografisk Tidsskrift.* Vol. 50. No 2, pp. 101-112.

This study is a review of current debates on fertility decline in Sub-Saharan Africa. The author argues that a new perspective on Africa's fertility situation is emerging, which differs from the old perspective as to why fertility was high in the region. The study argues that special attention be paid to the uniqueness of the African cultural setting in the quest for seeking explanations for the recent fertility change.

287. Agyei-Mensah, S. (1997). *Fertility Change in A Time and Space Perspective. Lessons From Three Ghanaian Settlements.* Ph.D Thesis Norwegian University of Science and Technology, Trondheim, Norway, 1997, 361 pages.

The study examines the evidence of fertility change in Ghana based on a time and space perspective. Time is operationalised by the use of a cohort model drawing on three birth cohorts of women born in the 1950s, 1960s and 1970s. To capture the spatial dimension, five distinct socio-economic areas are selected for the study. Different patterns of fertility change are observed based on area and birth cohort. The study also shows that the determinants of fertility change are to a large extent governed by the stage of the fertility transition at which the given society is.

288. Agyei-Mensah, S. (1997). A Scenario for fertility change in Sub-Saharan Africa up to 2020. *Bulletin of the Ghana Geographical Association,* Vol. 20, pp 101-116.

The author explores possible scenarios for fertility change in Sub-Saharan Africa by 2020. He first gives a review of fertility trends in Africa and then examines some of the factors underlying these changes. He then builds up the scenarios for the year 2020. Four scenarios are discussed: The replacement fertility scenario; the near replacement fertility scenario; the moderate fertility scenario; and the increasing, stabilizing, declining fertility scenario. The study concludes that given the diffferent fertility levels and background characteristics of countries and regions in Sub-Saharan Africa, one would not expect these countries and regions to follow a single uniform fertility pattern.

289. Agyei-Mensah, S. & A. Aase. (1997). *Patterns of Fertility Change in Ghana. A Time and Space Perspective.* (Unpublished manuscript.)

This paper examines fertility change in Ghana based on a time and space perspective. The sample draws on three birth cohorts of women born in the 1950s, 1960s and the 1970s, resident in five distinct societies selected from three settlements in the country. The findings of the study show that fertility change is occurring in a socio-economic and geographically distinct manner. Significant fertility declines are traced to the 1960s birth cohorts in all the study areas. For the 1970s cohort this decline continues in the elite areas whereas the urban indigenous areas exhibit a rise in teenage fertility, which is not, however, followed by higher fertility after the age of 20. In the rural area fertility rises from the 1960s to the 1970s cohort up to age 24, which is the end point of study for this cohort.

290. Ainsworth, M. (1988). Socio-economic determinants of fertility in Cote d'Ivoire. *Yale Economic Growth Center Discussion Paper 557,* July 28 pages.

This paper estimates a reduced form equation of the socio-economic determinants of fertility in Cote d' Ivoire. The study suggests among others that a fertility decline may be underway among the young educated women.

291. Anarfi, J. (1997). *Local herbs and fertility decline in Ghana: Contraceptives or as abortifacient?* Seminar presentation, Institute of Statistical, Social and Economic Research (ISSER), University of Ghana. 25th November 1997.

The most recent Ghana Demographic and Health Survey (GDHS, 1994) indicates that the Total Fertility Rate (TFR) has declined from 6.4 children per woman in 1988 to 5.5 in 1993, a decline of almost 1.0 in the five-year period. Within the same period, the rate of current use of contraception among currently married women increased from 13 percent to 20 percent. However, the current method mix of contraception is heavily tilted towards methods whose effectiveness level is suspect, abstinence and withdrawal. That implies that the current level of contraceptive prevalence and the method mix do not adequately account for the fertility decline that has been observed. What is the possible role of herbs in birth control in Ghana, and are they used as contraceptives or as abortifacient? This question is critically examined using information from existing literature and a pilot survey.

292. Ascadi, G.T.F, J. G. Ascadi, & R.A. Bulatao. (1990). *Population growth and reproduction in Sub-Saharan Africa. Technical analyses of fertility and its consequences.* World Bank Symposium 1990, 251 pages.

The papers presented here are edited and updated versions of background papers originally prepared for a 1983 World Bank policy study. They are divided into five sections. The demographic situation, economic consequences of rapid population growth, household and individual consequences of reproductive patterns, the context and causes of high fertility, and programs to reduce fertility. The aim of the volume is to bring together demographers findings about the nature and causes of Sub-Saharan Africa's population growth rate and economists findings about its implications.

293. Bankole, A. (1994). The role of mass media in family planning promotion in Nigeria. *DHS Working Paper, No. 11,* April 1994. 24 pages. Macro International, Demographic and Health Surveys (DHS), Calverton, Maryland.

The study provides an assessment of the role of mass media in the national task of promoting family planning and fertility decline. The question posed is: Does the Nigerian Demographic and Health Survey show the strong positive relationship between mass media and reproductive behaviour found in other DHS countries with similar data such as Kenya and Ghana among Sub-Saharan African countries?

294. Bankole, A. (1995). Desired Fertility and Fertility Behaviour among the Yoruba of Nigeria: A Study of Couple Preferences and Subsequent Fertility. *Population Studies*. 49 (2), pp. 317-28.

This paper examines the effects of fertility desires of marital partners on subsequent fertility. Specifically, it attempts to identify the role played by disagreement between spouses in predicting the couple's fertility outcome. The results indicate that when husband and wife disagree about whether or not they want another child, the fertility desires of both partners are equally important in determining whether the couple actually has an additional birth. The dominance of men in Sub-Saharan African societies tends to operate in the present study only in the initial stages of a couples reproductive lives (associated with four or fewer children). This tendency is offset by the stronger influence of the wives desire in the later stages. The study concludes that fertility research in Sub-Saharan Africa should solicit information from men and women, and any programme or policy that aims to promote fertility decline in the region must involve both sexes.

295. Bankole, A; G. Rodriguez; C. Westoff (1996). Mass media messages and reproductive behaviour in Nigeria. *Journal of Biosocial Science,* 28, pp. 227-239.

This paper examines the effects of exposure to mass media messages promoting family planning on the reproductive behaviour of married women in Nigeria using cross sectional data. Longitudinal data are also used to ensure that exposure to media messages pre-dates the indicators of reproductive behaviour. Cross sectional analyses suggests that contraceptive use and intention are positively associated with exposure to mass media messages, and women who are exposed to media messages are more likely to desire fewer children than those who are not exposed to such messages. Similarly, analysis of the longitudinal data shows that exposure to mass media messages is a significant predictor of contraceptive use. Thus exposure to mass media messages about family planning may be a powerful tool for influencing reproductive behaviour in Nigeria.

296. Barbieri, M. (1994). Is the current decline in infant and child mortality in Sub-Saharan Africa a sign of future fertility changes? In Locoh T. and V. Hertrich (eds.). *The Onset of Fertility Transition in Sub-saharan Africa.* pp 21-42. IUSSP, Liege. Belgium: Derouaux Ordina Editions.

The study seeks to determine whether Sub-Saharan Africa will follow the lead set by other countries. Will the reductions in infant and child mortality lead to a gradual lowering of fertility? It advocates a threshold level at which declines in infant mortality will lead to fertility declines at around 100 to 150 per thousand live births.

297. Barney, C. quoted in Caldwell, J.C. (1994). Fertility in Sub-Saharan Africa: Status and prospects. *Population and Development Review,* Vol. 20 no 1, pp. 179-187.

The author argues that substantial fertility decline has occurred in Zimbabwe, Kenya and Botswana, but since these countries account for only one-fifteenth of Africa's population, one cannot really tell of any appreciable fall in regional fertility in Africa.

298. Betrand, J.T.E, K. Bauni, R.J. Lesthaeghe, M.R. Montgomery, O. Tambashe, M.J. Wawer. (1993). *Factors Affecting Contraceptive Use in Sub-Saharan Africa.* National Research Council. National Academy Press. Washington D.C. 1993, 252 pages.

The main question posed in this book is whether Sub-Saharan Africa is on the brink of a contraceptive revolution that signals the onset of fertility decline. The findings of the study show that although there is considerable uncertainty about Africa as a whole, the evidence on balance points to an undeniable trend in Zimbabwe, Botswana, and Kenya. The changes observed in these three countries over the past decade indicate that selected parts of Africa have joined other regions of the developing world in a contraceptive revolution.

299. Benefo, K.D. & T.P. Schultz. (1994). Determinants of fertility and child mortality in Cote d'Ivoire and Ghana. *Living Standards Measurement Study Working Paper.* No. 103 May. 1994. 88 pages. World Bank, Washington D.C.

The author's explore the relationship between child mortality and fertility in Cote d'Ivoire and Ghana. They first discuss separately the reduced form determinants of fertility and child mortality, as explained by individual, household and community characteristics. Fertility is somewhat higher in Cote d'Ivoire than in Ghana and appears not to have changed recently in either country. Women's education beyond the primary level is associated with substantially lower fertility in both countries. The findings of the study suggest that Ghana is further along in its fertility transition than is Cote d'Ivoire.

300. Benneh, G., J.S. Nabila, J.S. Songsore, P.W.K. Yankson. (1990). *Demographic Studies and Final Projections for Accra Metropolitan Area* (AMA), UNDP, UNCHS, Ministry of Local Government, Accra.

The study examined among others the issue of fertility within the metropolis of Accra City, Ghana. They observed that there was an interest in small to medium sized families, which was generally shared by all income strata with few variations by class. By implication, they suggested that we are seeing a preference for smaller families over time.

301. Blacker, J. (1994). Some Thoughts on the Evidence of Fertility Decline in Eastern and Southern Africa; a review of National Research Council, Population Dynamics of Sub-Saharan Africa, *Population and Development Review,* 20 (1) pp. 200-205.

The study examines some of the problems involved in analysing data on fertility change in Sub-Saharan Africa. The emphasis is on the recent published reports from the National Academy of Sciences panel on population dynamics of Sub-Saharan Africa. The author raises serious issues with regards to sampling framework used for the Kenyan Demographic and Health Survey (KDHS). He argues that limitations regarding sampling is likely to affect the fertility estimates.

302. Blanc, A.K. & S. O. Rustein. (1994). The Demographic Transition in Southern Africa: Yet another look at the evidence from Botswana and Zimbabwe. *Demography,* Vol. 31, no 2, pp. 209-215.

The author's reach certain conclusions based on their analysis of the evidence of the decline in fertility in Botswana and Zimbabwe. Their argument hinges on the fact that there is no statistically significant difference in the distributions of women by educational status based on the 1984 and 1988 surveys.

303. Bradley, C. (1994). Declining fertility and wealth flows in Maragoli. In Thomas Weisner, Candice Bradley, and Philip Kilride (eds.), *African Families and the Crisis of Social Change.* Westport, CT: Greenwood Press.

The study examines the recent fertility decline in Kenya and the influence of wealth flows. It provides convincing evidence that fertility decline has begun in Kenya.

304. Bradley, C. (1995). Women's empowerment and fertility decline in Western Kenya. In Susan Greenhalgh (ed.). *Situating Fertility. Anthropology and Demographic Inquiry*. Cambridge University Press. pp. 157-178.

The study looks at the relationship between women's empowerment, domestic violence and fertility using data from Maragoli sub-location in Western Kenya. The author argues that though fertility is declining and contraceptive use is increasing in the area, these changes cannot be connected unproblematically to a single factor.

305. Brass, W. & C. Jolly. (Eds.). (1993). *Population Dynamics of Kenya.* Washington DC: National Academy Press.183 pages.

The study analyses Kenya's population dynamics with particular emphasis on recent fertility change. It is made up of eight chapters dealing with several aspects of the population of Kenya including her demography and socio-economic background, mortality trends, as well as fertility trends.

306. Brass, W. (1993). Child mortality improvement and the initiation of fertility falls in Kenya. *International Population Conference, Montreal 1993. Liege: IUSSP*, Vol. 1, pp. 73-80

The author explores the linkages between the fall in child mortality and fertility in Kenya. The conclusions of the study do not provide any consistent evidence that the declines in fertility were preceded by a fall in child mortality.

307. Brockerhoff, M. (1995). Fertility and family planning in African cities. The impact of female migration. *Journal of Biosocial Science*, 27, pp. 347-358.

The study shows that female migration from villages and towns in the 1980s and early 1990s reduced total fertility rates in African cities by about one birth per woman, from an estimated average of 5.5 in the absence of migration to 4.59.

308. Brockerhoff, M & M. Yang. (1994). The impact of migration on fertility in Sub-Saharan Africa. *Social Biology,* 41. pp. 19-43.

This article is based on data derived from DHS covering 6 countries Ghana, Kenya, Mali, Senegal, Togo and Uganda to examine the impact of long-term rural-urban female migration on fertility. The decline in fertility among the migrants is seen as a result of improvements in the standard of living experienced by migrants after settling in the urban area and may be due in part to temporal spousal separation.

309. Brown, G.F. (1991). An African challenge. Cut high fertility rate. *Forum for Applied Research and Public Policy*, 6 (2), pp. 31-35.

The study outlines some of the problems of the African landscape such as the high fertility rate, the rise in AIDS-related mortality, a long-term drought, political instability, widespread malnutrition, and periodic starvation. He argues that rapid population growth is an underlying factor that exacerbates this problem. In order to help arrest this situation, he suggests a reduction in the region's fertility rate.

310. Brunborg, H. (1990). A Brief Comparison of Recent Estimates of the Total Fertility Rate for Botswana. *Botswana Notes and Records* 20 Gaborone: Government Printer, pp. 91-98.

The author takes up the issue of fertility estimates of the 1971 and 1981 census data for Botswana and acknowledges that the two data sets are not fully comparable since somewhat different methods were used. He argues that ideally, the fertility rates for 1981 should have been estimated using the birth order data.

311. Buor, D. (1997). Pitfalls in fertility control in Ghana. *Journal of the University of Science and Technology,* Kumasi. Oct 1997.

The study examines the factors that inhibit the regulation of fertility in Ghana. The data is drawn from two districts in the Ashanti region of the country: Kwabre-Sekyere and Kumasi. Two factors are identified as inhibiting fertility control, illiteracy and outmoded customs.

312. Caldwell, J.C. (1965). Extended Family Obligations and Education: A Study of an aspect of Demographic Transition among Ghanaian University Students. *Population Studies*, Vol 19, no 2 pp 183-199.

This study sought to find out the evidence of fertility transition in Ghana. It is one of the earliest attempts at documenting the evidence of demographic change in Ghana.

313. Caldwell, J.C. (1968). *Population growth and family change in Africa. The new urban elite in Ghana*. Canberra, Australia National University Press, 213 pages.

The study looks at population growth and family change in Africa with a focus on the Ghanaian urban elite. Various aspects of demographic, family and attitudinal aspects were examined and related to aspects of the respondent's experience or behaviour. The study observed incipient fertility decline, socioeconomic and urban rural residence, fertility differentials and an inter relationship between private and public acceptance of population control. It attributed fertility transition among urban elite to declining family size due to delayed marriages and need and availability of extended training in towns.

314. Caldwell, J.C. & P. Caldwell (1978). The Achieved Small Family: Early Fertility Transition In An African City. *Studies in Family Planning,* Vol. 9, and No 1, pp. 2-18.

The paper is a report on a 1973 survey in Ibadan City, Nigeria, aimed at gathering information on deliberate fertility limitation in high fertility populations. The study found that both fertility decline and mortality decline are usually related to basic social changes involving the family, such as the shift to the child centered family.

315. Caldwell, P. & J.C. Caldwell (1987). Fertility Control as innovation. A report on in-depth interview in Ibadan, Nigeria. In *The Cultural roots of African fertility regimes*, pp. 233-251.

The main objective of the study was to obtain information from 1050 respondents who had never attempted to limit fertility by any means except sexual abstinence. It was evident that traditionally in the Yoruba society, postpartum abstinence was rigidly observed usually for a period of two to three years since this helped in shaping sexual practices and sexual mores of the society.

316. Caldwell, C., Caldwell, P., Orubuloye, I. (1992). Fertility decline in Africa: A new type of transition? *Population and Development Review,* 18, pp 211-242.

A number of recent surveys show that fertility has begun to decline in Botswana, Zimbabwe, Kenya, and Southern Nigeria. This article about an urban area in Southwest Nigeria confirms a fertility decline and throws light on the erosion of traditional supports for high fertility. The study concludes that the Sub-Saharan African fertility transition is likely to differ during its early decades from the pattern established by European and Asian transitions.

317. Caldwell, J.C. & P. Caldwell. (1987). The limitation of family size in Ibadan City, Nigeria. An explanation of the comparative rarity derived from in-depth interviews. In *The cultural roots of African fertility regimes*, proceedings of the Ife Conference, pp. 347-363.

The study looks at family limitation in Ibadan, Nigeria. In this society children are usually viewed as investments towards old age and those parents of large families do gain economic returns, and so profligacy would not result in poverty. However, some parents limit their family size in order to give their children continued education which can be very expensive, and when such education will prevent the family economic plans from achieving the desired success if the family is too large. All the same, most parents are of the view that they can have four or five children and still be able to educate them simply so that they can enter into professional employment. Even though there is a considerable decline in infant mortality, many parents fail to limit their families for fear of eventual childlessness. The study argues that there are strong cultural and religious practices, which work against the termination of reproduction in the Yoruba society, and these do not augur well for the achievement of fertility decline in Ibadan City.

318. Caldwell, J.C., Caldwell, P., Orubuloye, I. (1993). The South African fertility decline. *Population and Development Review,* 19 no 2 June, pp 225-262.

The study examines fertility decline in South Africa. With the publication of analyses based on household fertility surveys, patterns of demographic change in South Africa are now emerging. It is evident that each of the country's four racial groups has undergone demographic transitions, at different periods of time, with the black population displaying the most significant decline. The authors conclude that the decline has been prompted by the country's extensive family planning program, and it is suggested that similar declines in fertility could occur in other African nations if they were to adopt such vigorous programs as the South African one.

319. Caldwell, J.C. (1994). Fertility in Sub-Saharan Africa: Status and Prospects; review of National Research Council, Population Dynamics of Sub-Saharan Africa, *Population and Development Review,* Vol. 20 no 1 p 179-187:

The study discusses the recent publication of seven volumes on various aspects of demography in Sub-Saharan Africa. It concentrates on the debate as to whether there will be a general decline in fertility in Sub-Saharan Africa and whether the chief instrument in this decline will be a family planning program.

320. Campbell, E. & P.G. Campbell. (1997). Family Size and Sex preferences and eventual fertility in Botswana. *Journal of Biosocial Science.* 29, pp 191-204.

Botswana is one of the Sub-Saharan African countries where actual fertility has declined. This study examines the fertility preferences of both men and women and shows that fertility intentions have a significant influence on future fertility behaviour.

321. Campbell, E. (1994). Fertility, family size preferences and future fertility prospects of men in the western area of Sierra Leone. *Journal of Biosocial Science,* 26, 273-277.

Current fertility of men and women in the Western area of Sierra Leone and the prospects for future fertility behaviour are examined. Probably due to the effect of rapid economic decline in Sierra Leone since 1980, the desired family size has fallen. But indications are that the preferred completed family size is lower than the desired family size.

322. Chege, J.N (1993). *The politics of gender and fertility regulation in Kenya: A Case study of the Igembe.* Ph.D. Dissertation University of Lancaster UK.

The study looks at the role of gender relations in fertility regulation based on the experience of the Igembe of Kenya.

323. Chimere-Dan, O. (1993). Racial Patterns of Fertility Decline in South Africa. In *International Union for the Scientific Study of Population, International Population Conference,* Montreal 1993, Vol. 1. 1993. 43-51 pp. International Union for the Scientific Study of Population (IUSSP) Liege, Belgium pp 43-51.

The author examines fertility decline among the various racial groups in South Africa. Available data show that fertility is declining for blacks, coloureds, Indians and whites in South Africa. However, the timing and speed of fertility decline vary among these racial groups. This paper shows the context in which the racial groups maintained different patterns of transition decline with emphasis on possible reasons for the observed lag in fertility decline among blacks.

324. Chojnacka, H. (1995). The role of nuptiality in the demographic transition. The case of Africa. A conceptual essay *Genus,* 51, pp. 117-150.

The study explores the role of marriage in the recent fertility change in Africa.

325. Cleland, J., N. Onuoha, & I. N. Timaeus. (1994). Fertility Change in Sub-Saharan Africa. A review of the evidence. In Therese Locoh and Veronique Hertrich (eds.). *The Onset of fertility transition in Sub-Saharan Africa,* pp. 1-20.

This article provides a review of recent trends in fertility in Sub-Saharan Africa. It argues that the skepticism about prospects of the decline in fertility that was so prevalent until recently has lost its credibility. The study anticipates that in East and Southern Africa, fertility decline is likely to spread to further countries. In West and Central Africa, however, the outlook is more uncertain. Moreover one would not expect fertility to begin to fall in those countries afflicted by war, civil strife and other disasters.

326. Cochrane, S.H & S.M. Farid (1989). Fertility in Sub-Saharan Africa: Analysis and Explanation. *World Bank Discussion Paper No.43.* Washington, DC: The World Bank.

The study analyses the fertility situation in Sub-Saharan based largely from the results of the World Fertility Survey. Among countries in Sub-Saharan Africa that took part in the survey, Ghana is seen as having one of the best prospects for a future fertility decline.

327. Cohen, B. (1993). Fertility levels, differentials and trends. In Foote, K.A, Hill, K.H and Martin, L. (Eds). *Demographic Change in Sub-Saharan Africa.* Washington, DC: National Academy Press, pp. 8-67.

The study provides a summary of existing knowledge on fertility levels, trends and differentials in Sub-Saharan Africa based largely on the World Fertility Survey, which began in the 1970s, and the Demographic and Health Surveys conducted in the 1980s.

328. Cross A.R; W. Obungu; & P. Kizito (1991). Evidence of a transition to lower fertility in Kenya. *International Family Planning Perspectives,* Vol., 17. No 1, March, pp. 4 - 7.

This article uses the results of the KCPS and KDHS in analysing trends in fertility in Kenya. The study concludes that the transition to lower fertility has already begun and that increased use of family planning methods has been the major reason for the decline.

329. Dean, N.R. (1994). A community study of child spacing, fertility and contraception in West Pokot District, Kenya. *Social Science and Medicine,* Vol.38, No.11, June 1994. 1575-84 pp. Tarrytown, New York|Oxford, England.

Kenya is well known for its high fertility rate and West Pokot District has the highest population growth rate in Kenya. This study was designed to examine the community's perceptions of fertility dynamics. It looks at traditional methods of family planning and the recent changes in child spacing, fertility and contraception and attitudes behind them. This study also examines what the community (particularly women), want in the way of family planning services, The study used randomly selected groups throughout the district and employed a quasi-anthropological group discussion method.

330. Desta, Z. (1993*). The Population of Ethiopia, 1990-2025. Possibilities for the future.* Economics-Division Working Papers, Development Issues, Australian National University Research School of Pacific Studies, 34 pages.

Three future scenarios on the population of Ethiopia are provided in this study. The first scenario of the high variant projection assumes that the population would increase to 144 million by 2025, while the medium variant projects the population to grow to 125 million by 2025. The third scenario assumes that the population could be contained at about 110 million over the next 25 years.

331. Diamond, I. & N. Rutenberg. (1995). Recent trends in fertility in Botswana. *Journal of International Development.* 7 (1), pp. 145-161.

Fertility trends in Botswana have been the subject of much debate in recent years as a number of surveys in the mid to late 1980s suggested that a fertility decline was underway. This paper first reviews the demographic evidence for a fertility decline and argues that the magnitude of the decline was rather less than some commentators had suggested. The paper then places the trends in fertility in the social and economic context of Botswana in the 1980s. It is argued that there could have been a short-term decline in childbearing as a result of economic crises brought on by a major drought and helped by the government of Botswana's strategies to alleviate the effects of the drought on its people.

332. Diamond, I., & N. Rutenberg. (1993). Fertility in Botswana: The recent decline and future prospects. *Demography,* vol. 30 no 2, pp. 143-157.

The apparent simultaneous decline in fertility among rural and urban areas in Botswana forms a key issue in Rutenberg and Diamond's reaction to Botswana's fertility transition. They argue that the abrupt decline in the rural areas was a consequence of an economic crisis caused by the major drought that gripped the country for much of the 1980s.

333. Dodoo, F.N. (1993). A couple analysis of micro-level supply|demand factors in fertility regulation. *Population Research and Policy Review,* vol. 12, No. 2, pp. 93-101.

A joint- or couple-model is used to analyse fertility regulation in Ghana in order to illustrate the potential avenues that emerge when the input of male spouses is considered. The 1988 Ghana Demographic and Health Survey is used to examine the need for supply and demand side policy in achieving fertility declines. The results of the study shows that, although there is some evidence of the benefit of family planning programs, it appears that there is much room for further success. Also, there is a strong indication that the demand side of the fertility equation must be addressed more, by tackling the issue of individual motivations, particularly of males, for childbearing.

334. Dodoo, F. N. (1992). Female education, age, parity, and reproduction cessation in Ghana. *Social Biology,* Vol. 39, No. 1-2, pp. 102-108.

The study explores the relationship between education of the woman and her intention of ceasing childbearing in Ghana based on data derived from the 1988 DHS on Ghana. The findings of the study disagree with the view that people in Sub-Saharan Africa are not interested in fertility limitation. On the contrary educated people are interested though such desires are not translated into fertility decline.

335. Dodoo, F. N. (1993). Education and changing reproductive behaviour in Ghana. *Sociological Perspectives,* Vol. 36, No.3, autumn pp. 241-56. Greenwich, Connecticut.

Data from the 1988 Ghana Demographic and Health Survey is used to assess earlier speculation of fertility change in Ghana. The results of the study are cautiously optimistic. Although there is little evidence to support any hypothesis of a fertility turnaround in Ghana, there is some indication that continued increase in the proportion of women with some secondary education may yet induce a fertility transition in Ghana.

336. Dodoo, F.N. (1995). Contraceptive behaviour in Ghana: a two-sex model. *International Journal of Sociology of the Family,* Vol. 25, No 1, pp. 43-61.

The study uses DHS data on Ghana to examine the impact of male intentions on fertility related behaviour. The results of the study reveal that the reproductive preferences of male's spouses are not significant determinants of current use, although they may have some implications for future use. It is suggested that fertility may not have fallen in many parts of the region because men have not yet accepted a low fertility norm.

337. Dodoo, F.N. & A. Adomako Ampofo. (1997). *Report of the study on the Unmet Need of Men and Women in African Fertility Transition.* Rockefeller Foundation. 70 pages.

The study examines unmet need for men's and women's contraceptive behaviour with specific reference to the condom. The study is based on Demographic and Health Survey data drawn from Ghana and Kenya. Comparisons are made between urban and rural areas.

338. Douglas, R.M., G.W. Jones, R. M. D'Souza (eds.). (1996). The shaping of fertility and mortality declines. The contemporary demographic transition. *Health Transition Review* Supplement to volume 6, 1996, The Australian National University, Canberra, Australia, 396 pages.

This volume of the Health Transition series brings into perspective a collection of articles that touches on several aspects of demographic change particularly in Africa as well as other regions.

339. Dow, T. E. & L. H. Werner. (1983). Prospects for fertility decline in rural Kenya. *Population and Development Review,* 9, No. 1, pp. 77-97.

The study sought to examine the evidence of fertility decline in rural Kenya. The findings of the study revealed that neither economic nor emotional nucleation in rural Kenya was at a level sufficient to encourage the general acceptance of new fertility values and behaviour. The conclusion reached was that prospects for the early onset of fertility decline in rural areas were not promising.

340. Dow, T. E., L.Archer, S.Khasiani, & J.Kekovole. (1994). Wealth Flow and Fertility Decline in Rural Kenya 1981-1992, *Population and Development Review,* Vol. 20, pp. 343-364.

This article looked at the role of wealth flow in the decline in fertility in rural Kenya based on data collected in 1981 and 1992. The 1981 data did not find any evidence of fertility decline. Neither did it find any support for wealth flows. However, the 1992 study did find some evidence of fertility decline but limited evidence of economic or emotional nucleation within the household.

341. Dow, T.E, J. Kekovole, L. Archer. (1997). Wealth Flow and Fertility Decline in Rural Kenya, 1981-1992: A Reassessment of the Evidence. *African Journal of Reproductive Health,* Vol. 1, No 2, pp. 41-66.

This study is a re-assessment of data from studies conducted in Kenya in 1981 and 1992. The 1981 results showed a persistent high fertility with limited evidence of economic or emotional nucleation within the household. The 1992 survey however showed some evidence of fertility decline but nucleation levels were still the same. To resolve these issues a re-examination of the 1981 and 1992 data sets were made. The findings of the study showed the independent contribution of wealth flow and emotional nucleation variables.

342. Dzekedzeke, K. & N. Nelson. (1994). Fertility patterns and their determinants in Zambia: findings from the Zambia Demographic and Health Survey. In *DHS Regional Analysis Workshop for Anglophone Africa: fertility trends and determinants in six African countries.* April 1994. pp. 145-79, Calverton, Maryland.

Fertility trends and determinants in Zambia are assessed based on data from the 1992 Zambian Demographic and Health Survey. The study also explores the transitions to motherhood and first marriage, as well as fertility regulation and preferences.

343. Economist (1993). Why Africans want fewer babies? *Economist,* Jan. 1993.

The January 1993 edition of the Economist magazine reported of the evidence of fertility decline in Africa stressing why Africans want fewer babies.

344. Egero, B. & E. Mburugu. (1994). Kenya: reproductive change under strain. In: *Understanding reproductive change: Kenya, Tamil Nadu, Punjab, Costa Rica,* edited by B. Egero and M. Hammaskjold. 1994. 31-64 pages. Lund University Press, Lund, Sweden.

The study examines the roots of Kenya's high fertility regime in disruptions of pre-colonial family systems and social regulations of reproduction, and finds evidence that recent increases in birth control signify primarily a recapture of earlier birth-spacing patterns, and for older women, also an end to childbearing. The author's analyse the significance of women's growing awareness of and ability to adjust their reproduction in response to increasing constraints through land shortage, unemployment, and costs for schooling and other services.

345. Ekouevi K & A. Adepoju. (1995). Adjustment, social sectors, and demographic change in Sub-Saharan Africa. *Journal of International Development,* 7 (1) pp. 47-59.

The effects of the structural adjustment policies on fertility change in Sub-Saharan Africa are analysed. Two speculative scenarios are made with regards to the future prospects of the decline. One, is a delayed transition with the persistence of factors that sustain high fertility, and the other, a crisis led transition where economic hardship might accelerate the decline.

346. Fairlamb, C. D. & W. L. Nieuwoudt. (1991). Economic factors affecting human fertility in the developing areas of Southern Africa. *Agricultural Economics,* 6(2) pp. 185-200.

Economic factors explaining family size choice in the traditional sector were examined and linkages between family size decisions and socio-economic variables analysed. Results show that wives education, child help benefits and desired family size were important explanatory variables. Three components extracted represented the substitution effect, the income effect and child investment theory. Results show that investment in education, taken as a proxy for expected earnings, is a strong policy option for reducing family size.

347. Farooq, G.M. & L. A. Adeokun. (1976). Impact of a rural family planning program in Ishan, Nigeria, 1969-1972. *Studies in Family Planning,* 7, 6, pp. 158-169.

The Ishan pilot study in Nigeria reports on changes in proportions of women wanting no more children, although increasing contraceptive use, not decreasing fertility preferences, was the primary objective.

348. Frank, O. & J. Bongaarts. (1991). Behavioural and Biological determinants

of fertility transition in Sub-Saharan Africa. *Statistics in Medicine*. Vol. 10, pp. 161-195.

The author examines the behavioural and biological determinants of fertility transition in Sub-Saharan Africa and argues that a transition to low fertility would come with a substantial increase in modern contraception.

349. Gaisie, S.K. (1996). Demographic transition: the predicament of Sub-Saharan Africa. *Health Transition Review Supplement* to Volume 6, pp. 345-69. Canberra, Australia.

The author explores the peculiarities of Sub-Saharan Africa's demographic transition in light of changes in mortality, infrastructure and fertility. He argues for the importance of historical, cultural and international economy in our understanding of the observed trends.

350. Goldberg, H.I; M. McNeil; A. Spitz. (1989). Contraceptive use and fertility decline in Chogoria, Kenya. *Studies in Family Planning*, 20 (1). pp. 17-25.

This article describes the results pertaining to fertility and family planning from a 1985 survey conducted in the catchment area of Chogoria hospital in Central Kenya. Current contraceptive prevalence was found to be quite high, 43 percent as opposed to 17 percent for Kenya as a whole. The TFR of 5.2 births per woman was 2.5 births lower than the national rate.

351. Gould, W.T.S. (1995). Ideology and data analysis in African population policies: the case of Kenya. *Applied Geography*, 15 (3), pp. 203-218.

Formal population policies are now common in Sub-Saharan Africa, particularly to directly facilitate fertility decline. They tend to be underpinned more by ideology than by systematic data collection and analysis. A case study of policies to promote fertility decline in Kenya where fertility has fallen substantially in recent years illustrates how population data, particularly from the 1989 and 1993 DHS have been used by government and international agencies to validate than to inform official policy.

352. Guilkey, D. & S. Jayne. (1997). Fertility transition in Zimbabwe: Determinants of contraceptive use and method choice. *Population Studies*. pp. 173-189.

A structural equation model is used to assess the determinants of contraceptive method choice in Zimbabwe. The data is based on the 1989 Zimbabwe Demographic and Health Survey. The findings of the study show that wives education; husbands education, family planning messages, and the presence of a community based distributor of contraceptives have contributed to Zimbabwe's highly successful family planning programme.

353. Gule, G. (1994). A Review of family planning in Sub-Saharan Africa. *African Population Paper,* No.2, Aug 1994. 27 pages. African Population and Environment Institute, Nairobi, Kenya.

The study provides a review of family planning in Sub-Saharan Africa. Pockets of fertility decline are observed even though the region still has the highest fertility rate in the world. For most countries of the region, the total fertility rate is generally above 6, knowledge of contraceptives is much higher than its use, and in the countries with rising contraceptive prevalence rates, fertility decline is already taking place. It is concluded that the four countries where fertility transition has occurred namely Zimbabwe, Botswana, South Africa and Kenya are the countries that have successful family planning programmes, in the last country supported by a long standing population policy.

354. Hailemariam, A. (1991). Fertility levels and trends in Arsi and Shoa regions of Central Ethiopia. *Journal of Biosocial Science,* Oct 23 (4) Page 387-400.

Levels and trends of fertility in the Arsi and Shoa regions of Central Ethiopia are examined, using data from the 1986 Population, Health and Nutrition baseline survey of the Ministry of Health of Ethiopia. The population has high fertility. Total Fertility of six children per woman in the late 1960s increased to eight children per woman in the early 1980s, then declined to seven children per woman in the mid-1980s. Urban fertility declined by a substantial amount during the 15 years before the survey while rural fertility increased during the same period. The implications of high fertility are considered.

355. Hammerslough, C. R (1992). Proximity to contraceptive services and fertility transition in rural Kenya. *International Family Planning Perspectives.* vol. 18 no. 2, June.

The role of contraceptives in Kenya's fertility decline forms a central theme in the author's study. Based on a multivariate analysis he reaches the conclusion that increased contraceptive services accelerated Kenya's transition but it did not initiate the transition. Family planning availability he notes is a necessary but insufficient condition for modern fertility transitions in Sub-Saharan Africa.

356. Harbison, S.F & W. C. Robinson. (1993). Components of The Recent Fertility Decline In Kenya. *Population Research Institute Working Paper no. 1993- 06.* Pennsylvania State University.

The study examines the components of Kenya's recent fertility decline, and looks at the interaction of supply and demand factors, which have contributed to the decline. It argues that family planning can work in Sub-Saharan Africa when an effective service delivery program is put in place and sufficient socio-economic change occurs to stimulate changes in values and attitudes towards fertility.

357. Hill, K.H; G. Adansi-Pipim; L. Assogba; A. Foster; J. Mukiza-Gapere; C.H. Paxson. (1993). *Demographic Effects of the Economic Reversals in Sub-Saharan Africa*, 193 pages. Washington, DC: National Academy Press.

This study examines the effects of economic reversals on recent fertility change in Sub-Saharan Africa. The findings of the study does not give any strong claim that economic crisis is affecting fertility decline.

358. Institute of Resource Development. (IRD). Sharp Drop in Fertility Seen in Latest Ghana Survey. *Demographic and Health Surveys Newsletter* (1996) vol. 8. No 1. pp 5.

This edition of the IRD Newsletter provides information on Ghana's recent fertility decline and argues that the sharp decline in fertility is associated with an increased use of modern contraceptive methods.

359. Isiugo-Abanihe, U.C. (1994). Reproductive motivation and family size preferences among Nigerian men. *Studies in Family Planning,* 25 (3) pp 149-61.

This study examines reproductive decision making and male motivation for large families in five Nigerian settlements. It concludes that dominant male and patrilineal traditions encourage large family sizes and that to a large extent, men's reproductive motivation determines that of their wives. The study of factors influencing men's reproductive behaviour is therefore important in the understanding of fertility change in Nigeria.

360. Jensen, A.M. & M.N. Yuma. (1989). *Women, Childbearing and Nutrition. A case study from Bungoma, Kenya*. Norwegian Institute for Urban and Regional Research, Oslo. 293 pages.

The study looks at the inter relation between the situation of women, fertility patterns and nutrition education in Bungoma, Western Kenya. The report comprises two studies: childbearing and nutrition education. It consists of four sections. Section 1 is background information, which relates to both studies. Section 2 is on the situation of women and childbearing. Section 3 is on nutrition education. Section 4 gives recommendations, which are based on experiences from both studies. Women living in sub-locations with a higher dependency of money economy had lower number of children. The most urbanised area with lowest fertility also had the lowest child mortality. However, also in the most modern sublocation 45 percent of the women had lost a child, which indicates that other factors at a social level also are important in explaining a lower number of children in modern areas.

361. Jensen, A.M. (1991). Economic change, marriage relations and fertility in a rural area of Kenya. In *Gender and change in developing countries,* edited by Kristi A. Stolen and Mariken Vaa. 1991. pp 67-89. Norwegian University Press, Oslo, Norway.

This is an analysis of fertility in Bungoma District, a rural area of Kenya located near the Ugandan border, a region of high fertility and low contraceptive practice. Data were collected through interviews of 65 women in 1988. The focus of the analysis is on linkages between social change and adjustments at the family level, especially on changes in marital patterns and in infant mortality. The author concludes that there have been changes in the perceived value of children, particularly among nuclear families, but that although family planning concepts were known they were not applied, primarily because infant and child mortality levels had not yet been reduced sufficiently for parents to be sure of having living children to support them in old age.

362. Jensen, A.M. (1995). The status of women and the social context of reproduction. *Journal of International Development.* 7 (1), pp 61-79.

The aim of this article is to broaden the understanding of the uneven pace of fertility decline in Kenya. The data is based upon two case studies, from Kwale in coast province and Bugoma in the western province. Attention is given to the social value of children and the role of women.

363. Jensen, A.M. (1993). Child Survival and Fertility in Kenya. *Forum for Development Studies* (NUPI). No 1 pp 37-47. Oslo, Norway.

This study examines the interplay between child survival, fertility and acceptance of family planning based on Kenya. The discussion begins at the aggregate level where regional differences are discussed. The last section focuses on the individual level, discussing fertility and family planning among women who have, or have not, experienced the loss of a child. In this section data from case studies on two areas with a high level of child mortality are employed, Western and Coast. The two areas differ in terms of fertility levels. While fertility rates in Western province are at high levels, Coast province has relatively low fertility. The paper reveals that fertility in both areas is higher among women who have lost a child. The low fertility in Coast reflects that many women in this area suffer from subfecundity. Both child loss and subfecundity has a negative impact on use of modern contraceptives.

364. Jensen, A.M. (1996). *Fertility-Between the Passion and Utility. The Value of children and demographic changes.* Dr. Polit. thesis. The Department of Sociology and Human Geography, University of Oslo.

This work is a collection of articles on fertility change mainly drawn from Kenya. It was submitted for the author's doctoral degree. The main thesis here is that the value of children is an important determinant of fertility. Where children do not have a high social value, there is less need to control their birth and women have more independence.

365. Jensen, A.M. (1995). Prospect of a Decline in Fertility in Sub-Saharan Africa: A Review of the Recent Debate. *Acta Sociologica,* 38, pp 263-273.

The author examines the current debate on fertility transition in Africa using Kenya as a case study. She argues that the prospects for a decline are still not clear in Kenya given the fact that Kenyan women have more than five children during their lifetime, and children still represent security in old age.

366. Jensen, A.M. (1995). Is there a link between Fertility Decline and Family Planning in Kenya? In C. Lundh (ed.). *Demography, Economy and Welfare, Scandinavian Population Studies* 10 pp 351-365.

The study examines Kenya's fertility decline and links the decline to modern contraceptive uptake.

367. Jensen, A. M. & A. A. Khasakhala. (1992). Women, family planning and child mortality. Case study of selected areas in Kenya, Western and Coast provinces. In A. Manu (eds.). *Health and Environment in Developing Countries.* Proceedings of international workshop, Lovlia, 1991 University of Oslo Center for Development and the Environment pp 19-42.

This paper examines the interplay between fertility, family planning and child mortality. Empirical examples are drawn from Kenya, a country with one of the highest fertility rates in the world. Two communities in the Bungoma and Kwale districts, with differing socio-economic statuses and religious inclinations offer possible explanations to the dynamics of demographic behaviour. The trend is that low fertility seems to be related to cash economy, high education, less men domination, and quite surprisingly, high marriage instability.

368. Journal of International Development (1995). Vol. 17, No. (1).

This issue of the Journal of International Development is devoted to the emerging fertility transition in Sub-Saharan Africa. The focus is on development change and fertility decline.

369. Jones, H. (1989). Fertility decline in Mauritius. The role of Malthusian population pressure. *Geoforum,* 20 (3) pp 315-327.

Mauritius provides one of the outstanding cases of modern fertility reduction in the third world, yet there has been little analysis and virtually no comparative assessment of its important demographic progression. The study argues that fertility decline in Mauritius has been hindered by cultural composition, but aided significantly by family planning programme intervention and by a remarkably wide recognition at government and individual mlebels of the diseconomies associated with population growth in the congested society.

370. Kalipeni, E. (1995). Fertility transition in Africa. *Geographical Review.* 85 (2) pp 287-30.

The fertility transition in Africa is examined. It is argued that fertility transition is largely believed to be due to worsening environmental and economic conditions rather than due to the influences of modernisation per se.

371. Kalipeni, E. (1996). Demographic Response to Environmental Pressure in Malawi. *Population and Environment,* 17, (4) pp 285-308.

The study examines the interrelationship between population growth and demographic responses to environmental pressure, using Malawi as a case study. The study reveals that parts of Malawi experiencing extreme environmental stress have begun a rapid phase of demographic and social transformation. For example the southern region of the country, which has some of the highest population densities, is experiencing a fertility transition.

372. Kalipeni, E. (1997). Population Pressure, Social Change, Culture and Malawi's Pattern of Fertility Transition. *African Studies Review,* Volume 40, Number 2. pp. 173-208.

Fertility rates in Malawi continue to be among the highest in the world, while mortality rates have declined significantly. This study uses crude birth rates and total fertility rates in examining the spatial context of fertility in Malawi. The results indicate that at the regional and district levels, fertility rates are associated with the spatial variation of certain factors of modernisation and cultural practices that have a direct bearing on child spacing such as infant mortality rates, age at first marriage, population density, females in non-agricultural occupations and kinship system. The results of the study seem to indicate that rural areas experiencing high population pressures will be among the first areas to initiate a fertility transition.

373. Kelley, A.C, Nobbe, C.E. (1990). Kenya at the demographic turning point?

Hypothesis and a proposed agenda. *World Bank Discussion Papers, no. 107,* Washington, D.C: World Bank, pp xvi, 97.

The study examines the record of population change in Kenya and discusses how the Kenyan economy has performed, accommodated and been influenced by rapid population growth.

374. Kidane, A. (1985). Economic Growth and the demographic transition: the case of African countries. *African Review,* 12 (2) Page 77-88.

The author outlines the theory of demographic transition, and discusses its shortcomings and relevance to present day developing countries. The paper attempts to empirically verify the relevance of the theory to African countries, specifically studying the extent to which the socio-economic performances of the past twenty years have decreased mortality and fertility rates

375. Kisanje, M. & J.K. Kalule. (1994). The estimation of potential demand for contraception and the implication for fertility in Uganda. In *DHS Regional Analysis Workshop for Anglophone Africa: fertility trends and determinants in six African countries.* April 1994. pp 121-43. Calverton, Maryland.

Data from the 1988-89 Ugandan Demographic and Health Survey are used to examine fertility levels and determinants. The study also discusses the existing demand for family planning and on that basis make estimates of the appropriate contraceptive method mix that would be required to meet the current demand of contraception in Uganda.

376. Kizito, P., W. Obungu, M. Kibet, W. Njogu. (1991). Fertility transition in Kenya. *DHS Further Analysis Studies,* No. 11. Dec 1991 23 pages. Macro International, Demographic and Health Surveys. Calverton. Maryland.

Fertility change in Kenya is examined within the proximate determinant framework. The study is based on three main objectives. The first one is to describe fertility levels and trends at the aggregate and subgroup level, classified by level of education and type and region of residence. The second objective is to document trends in the proximate determinants of fertility (breast feeding, contraceptive use, marital patterns, postpartum infecundability and sterility). The third objective is to examine the relative role of the various determinants of the fertility decline

377. Kojima, H. (1994). Effects of mass media on contraception and fertility in African countries. In S. Kono & Y. Hayase (eds.). *Fertility in the developing Countries. A comparative study of the Demographic and Health Surveys.* IDE Statistical Data Series No. 66. Institute of Developing Economies, Tokyo, Japan. pp 133-180.

The study explores the effects of two variables specifically related to radio on contraception and fertility in five African countries for which information on these variables is available. They are household's possession of a radio and the wives exposure to family planning messages on the radio. The results of the study suggest that both socio-economic development policies and family planning programs with a special emphasis on mass media; especially radio may have significant effects on fertility control in developing countries. The results also suggest that the free or subsidised distribution of a radio among households could lead to socio-economic development with controlled fertility even without family planning campaigns on the radio.

378. Komba, A. & C. L. Kamuzora. (1988). Fertility reduction due to non-marriage and lactation. A case study of Kibaha district, Tanzania. In *African Population Conference, Dakar, vol. 1.* 2.1.53-2.1.71

A survey was carried out in 1986 in the Kibaha District in the coast region of Tanzania to measure the effects of non-marriage and post partum infecundability to the high level of fertility in the region. Using Bongaarts (1978) model, the study found that the combined effect of non-marriage and infecundability reduces fertility.

379. Lesthaeghe, R. J. & C. Jolly. (1995). The Start of the Sub-Saharan fertility transition: some answers and many questions. *Journal of International Development* 7 (1) pp 25-45:

The author's examine the possible factors underlying the recent fertility change in Sub-Saharan Africa. They argue that while the theory of the crisis led fertility transition can help explain this outcome, the theory also has its limitations. If the crisis deepens and hits the health and education sectors, negative effects emerge as crucial props such as female schooling levels and family planning provisions may suffer adverse set backs.

380. Letamo, G. (1996). Contributions of the proximate determinants to fertility change in Botswana. *Journal of Biosocial Science,* 28, pp 325-338.

The proximate determinants framework as advanced by Bongaarts is used to examine the relative contributions of the three proximate determinants, non marriage, contraceptive use and postpartum infecundability to fertility change using data from the 1984 and 1998 Botswana Family and Health Surveys. Breast-feeding is shown to be the most important proximate determinant of fertility, followed by contraceptive use, and finally nonmarriage, both in 1984 and 1988. However, contraceptive use increased between 1984 and 1988, leading to fertility decline over this period. Marriage is the least important proximate determinant of fertility, probably due to the high prevalence of premarital childbearing. Other factors such as induced abortion could have played a major role in fertility decline but their effect could not be estimated due to lack of accurate data.

381. Lockwood, M. (1995). Development Policy and the African Demographic Transition: Issues and Questions. *Journal of International Development.* 7 (1) pp 1-23.

This article examines the recent evidence of fertility decline in Sub-Saharan Africa. The author begins by providing evidence of the decline. He then goes on to provide explanations for the decline. The conclusion reached in the study is that despite an ever growing body of data on African demography and a range of theories on demographic change much is still unclear. It is recommended that micro level studies should be undertaken to complement the macro level data sets.

382. Locoh, T. (1994). Will the decline in fertility in Sub-Saharan Africa last? A time of uncertainty. In Therese Locoh and Veronique Hertrich (eds.). *The Onset of Fertility Transition in Sub-Saharan Africa.* International Union for the Scientific Study of Population (IUSSP). pp 105-133.

Against the background of recent declines in fertility in some African countries, the author looks at the stability in high fertility level in most of the countries based on data from Ghana, Togo and Rwanda. Analysis of data from these countries does not show that fertility levels that are stable on average. The study argues that the next 25 years will see the dawn of fertility transition in Sub-Saharan Africa. The transition, the study argues will adopt varied routes, including temporary increases in certain regions and in certain countries. To assist the transition it is further argued that our tools of analysis and diagnosis must be honed further, not only at a national level but also at the level of each socio-economic sub-group.

383. Locoh, T & V. Hertrich (Eds.) (1994). *The Onset of fertility transition in Sub-Saharan Africa.* International Union for the Scientific Study of Population-Liege: Derouaux Ordina Editions 308 pages.

This book contains articles emanating from the IUSSP conference in Harare in 1991. It contains a number of articles on fertility transition in Sub-Saharan Africa.

384. Loyola, R.B. (1992). *A general equilibrium model of the demographic transition in Sub-Saharan Africa.* PhD Dissertation University of Alberta, 1992, 402 pages.

A simulation model developed primarily using data for Kenya is used to assess the policy implications of projected demographic trends in Sub-Saharan Africa up to the year 2000.

385. Lucas, D. (1991). Mass education and fertility decline: implications for Southern Africa. Paper presented to the Seminar on the *Course of Fertility Transition in Sub-Saharan Africa,* sponsored by IUSSP Committee on Comparative Analysis of Fertility and the University of Zimbabwe, Harare, November 19-22.

The study examines the influence of mass education on fertility decline looking at the evidence from Southern Africa.

386. Lucas, D. (1992). Fertility and family planning in Southern and Central Africa. *Studies in Family Planning,* vol., 23, No.3, May-June 1992. pp 145-58. New York, New York.

Southern Africa is a region where TFRs is below 6 births per woman. To the north is a ring of countries with higher fertility and relatively low contraceptive prevalence rates. This article attempts to identify some reasons why Southern Africa has begun its fertility transition while Central Africa has not.

387. Macro International. Demographic and Health Surveys (DHS) (1994). *DHS Regional Analysis Workshop for Anglophone Africa: fertility trends and determinants in six African countries.* 215 pages, Calverton, Maryland.

This volume contains papers on fertility patterns in six-sub-Saharan African countries. The papers were written by participants in the 1992 Demographic and Health Surveys Program (DHS) Regional Analysis Workshop for Anglophone Africa. The primary objective of the workshop were for participants to carry out an analysis of the course of fertility and its determinants in their countries, to interpret this evidence in the context of the policy and socio-economic environment, and to identify and explore in depth fertility-related topics of particular policy or program relevance.

388. Makinwa-Adebusoye, P. (1994). Changes in the costs and benefits of children to their parents. In *The Onset of fertility transition in Sub-Saharan Africa.* Edited by Locoh, T. and V. Hertrich, 1994. pp 75-92. IUSSP, Liege. Belgium: Derouaux Ordina Editions.

This paper examines recent increases in child-rearing costs such as the costs of education, and their effects on the value of children in countries of sub-Saharan Africa. The first section reviews the main theoretical perspectives concerning the relationship between fertility and the costs and benefits of children. These theoretical perspectives are then discussed in the context of Sub-Saharan Africa. Parental aspirations for children's schooling and perceived attendant costs under conditions of economic hardship are examined.

389. Makinwa-Adebusoye, P.K, & B.J. Feyisetan. (1994). The quantum and tempo

of fertility in Nigeria. In: *DHS Regional Analysis Workshop for Anglophone Africa: fertility trends and determinants in six African countries,* April 1994. 41-86 pages. Calverton.

The study looks at fertility trends and determinants in Nigeria, based on the 1990 Nigeria Demographic and Health Survey. The author's first assess the quality of data from the survey questionnaires. They then briefly describe the characteristics of the women surveyed. Fertility levels and trends are examined, and finally fertility regulation and reproductive preferences are analysed.

390. Mazur, R.E & M. Mhloyi. (1994). Women's work and fertility in Zimbabwe: ending underdevelopment with change. In *Gender, Work and Population in Sub-Saharan Africa*, (ed.). By A. Adepoju and C. Oppong. 1994. pp. 132-56. James Currey, London, England.

The main objective of this paper is to improve understanding of the nature of the relationships between women's work and fertility in contemporary Zimbabwe. Having achieved independence in 1980, Zimbabweans find themselves in an era of rapid social and economic change. The available evidence concerning the structure of the economy and the nature of economic activity is first examined, with an emphasis on women's complex patterns of involvement. After a brief look at demographic trends in Zimbabwe, the relationship between women's economic activities and status and fertility patterns and differentials in Zimbabwe is compared with that observed in other societies.

391. Mbacke, C. (1994). Family planning programs and fertility transition in Sub-Saharan Africa; review of National Research Council, *Population Dynamics of Sub-Saharan Africa,* 20 no 1 pp188-193.

The author comments on the publication of Population Dynamics of Sub-Saharan Africa, a seven-volume set resulting from the work of a panel appointed by the National Academy of Sciences in 1989. He argues that the pessimism about the possibility of significant and rapid fertility decline in Sub-Saharan Africa that characterises much demographic research is a reflection of the inadequacy of the general framework of demographic theory for analysing demographic change in Africa.

392. Mhloyi, M.M. (1988). *The Determinants of fertility in Africa under modernisation.* In African Population Conference, Dakar vol. 1. 2.3.1 to 2.3.22.

Fertility in Africa has been very high due to certain factors deeply entrenched in the socio-cultural and economic fabric of the societies. It is recognised now that education and urbanisation are going to play a tremendous role in Africa's transition.

393. Mhloyi, M.M. (1994). Fertility Transition in Zimbabwe. In Locoh, T. and V. Hertrich (Eds). *The Onset of Fertility Transition in Sub-Saharan Africa.* International Union for the Scientific Study of Population pp 87-104.

The objective of the paper is to understand factors underlying fertility decline in Zimbabwe during the 20-year period 1969 to 1988. The study argues that the fertility transition in Zimbabwe has been a function of the changes both intended and unintended in the socio-economic factors that underlie fertility determinants.

394. Mturi, A.J. & P.R.A. Hinde (1995). Recent demographic change in Tanzania: causes, consequences and future prospects. *Journal of International Development.* 7 (1), pp 117-134.

The recent fertility decline in Tanzania is examined. The study shows a decline in fertility from seven children per woman in the early 1980s to about six in the early 1990s. The study argues that this trend is a result of a rise in the age at first marriage for women, a decline in infant and child mortality, a rise in the percentage of the population with education, and rural development. The continuing universal and prolonged breast-feeding also has a significant negative effect on fertility. A further fertility decline in Tanzania will depend mainly on the success of the family planning programme, which in turn will improve the performance of the economy, health, education, employment, agriculture and the environment. Mortality levels have declined but are still high owing to various factors including short birth intervals, teenage pregnancies, the low status of women, the lack of adequate health services, and a lack of proper programmes targeted at regions and families with relatively high mortality.

395. Mturi, A. J. & P.R.A. Hinde. (1994). Fertility Decline in Tanzania. *Journal of Biosocial Science,* 26, pp 529-538.

The paper analyses the social and demographic determinants of fertility in Tanzania based on the results of the 1991/1992 Tanzania Demographic and Health Survey. It shows that infant and child mortality, level of education and age at first marriage are the major factors, which influence fertility in Tanzania.

396. Muganzi, Z. & T. Timothy. (1994). Fertility decline and demand for family planning in Kenya. In *DHS Regional Analysis Workshop for Anglophone Africa: fertility trends and determinants in six African countries.* Calverton, Maryland, April 1994. 1-39 pages.

The recent fertility decline in Kenya is discussed in light of awareness, approval, and practice of family planning. The data is based on the 1989 Kenyan Demographic and Health Survey.

397. Muhwava, W.B., & I. Muvandi. (1994). Breast-feeding, contraceptive use, and fertility in Zimbabwe: a further analysis of the Demographic and Health Survey. In: *DHS Regional Analysis Workshop for Anglophone Africa: Fertility trends and determinants in six African countries.* April 1994. 181-215 pages. Calverton, Maryland.

The study had the following objectives: to document recent fertility trends in Zimbabwe, to make an analysis of trends and subnational fertility differentials using the data from the Zimbabwean Demographic and Health Survey (ZDHS), to show the policy implications of fertility trends, to analyse the proximate determinants of fertility in Zimbabwe, to assess the effect of socio-economic variables on fertility, and to examine the relationship between fertility and breastfeeding.

398. National Council for Population and Development (NCPD) (1989). *Kenya Demographic and Health Survey 1988.* Nairobi. Central Bureau of Statistics.

This report presents the first-ever significant decline in fertility in Kenya based on the demographic survey conducted in 1988.

399. National Council for Population and Development (Nairobi, Kenya). Kenya. Kenya Central Bureau of Statistics (Nairobi, Kenya) Macro International. Demographic and Health Surveys (DHS) Calverton, Maryland. (1994). *Kenya Demographic and Health Survey, 1993,* May 1994, 278 pages Nairobi, Kenya.

Results are presented from the second national demographic and health survey conducted in Kenya. This survey, carried out in 1993, involved a nationally representative sample of 7540 women aged 15-49 and 2336 men aged 20-54. The results reinforce evidence of a major decline in fertility, which was revealed by the findings of the 1989 survey. Fertility continues to decline and family planning use has increased. However, the disparity between knowledge and use of family planning remains quite wide. There are indications that infant and under five child mortality rates are increasing, which in part might be attributed to the increase in AIDS prevalence.

400. New York Times International. (1989). Birth control-making inroads in populous Kenya. *New York Times,* Sunday, 10 September.

This September edition of the New York Times came up with a story that fertility transition had begun in Kenya.

401. Ngom, P. (1997). Men's Unmet need for family Planning: Implications for African Fertility Transitions. *Studies in Family Planning,* Vol. 28, and No. 5 pp 192-202.

This article introduces the concept of men's unmet need for family planning and explains its programmatic relevance. The study is based on data from Demographic and Health Surveys (DHS) of Ghana (1988, 1993) and Kenya (1989, 1993). Married men are found to have high levels of unmet need for family planning that is comparable to, although slightly lower than, those for women. The importance of men's unmet need is demonstrated when the analysis is restricted to marital pairs in the DHS samples, trends in the joint unmet need of husbands and wives are shown to be closely associated with the nature of the fertility transitions occurring in Ghana and Kenya. The study concludes that because of the wide discrepancies found between husband's and wives unmet need statuses, family planning programs that foster spousal communication are likely to facilitate the transition to lower fertility.

402. Njogu, W. (1991). Trends and Determinants of Contraceptive use in Kenya. *Demography,* 28, pp 83-99.

Based on a comparison of the 1977/1978 Kenyan Fertility Survey and the 1989 Kenyan Demographic and Health Survey, the author observes that the percentage of contraceptive use (modern and traditional) among currently married women of reproductive age increased for all categories of each of the following demographic groups: reproductive age, desire for additional children, child loss experience, type of marital union, type and region of residence and educational level. The study shows that contraceptive use is not limited to older women who may have already given birth to a large number of children, but also more educated women and women residing in urban areas. It appears that a broad fertility reduction infrastructure is forming which should enable Kenya to attain further fertility reductions.

403. Njogu, W. & C.T. Martin. (1992). Fertility decline in Kenya: The role of timing and spacing of births. In *International Union for the Scientific Study of Population Seminar on Fertility Transition in Sub-Saharan Africa Harare, Zimbabwe,* 19-22 November 1991.

The authors examine Kenya's fertility decline and reveal that later age of marriage as observed in the 1989 KDHS has a negligible impact on fertility levels. Their conclusion is based on the fact that Kenyan women get married during the first pregnancy or after the first birth of the first child. Thus the high incidence of premarital births and conceptions shows that the date of first marriage is a poor indicator of the onset of sexual activity and hence of the exposure to childbearing.

404. Nkrumah, M. (1993). *Prospects for fertility decline in rural Southern Ghana. A case study of Amosima area.* Masters Thesis Dept of Geography University of Cape Coast Ghana. 187 pages.

The study examines Caldwell's intergenerational transfer of resources hypotheses as a factor leading to fertility decline in the Amosima area in Southern Ghana. The study reveals the existence of inter and intra-generational transfer of resources in the area. Specifically, four main types of transfer of resources are identified; parent to child, child to parent, among siblings and among matrikins.

405. Odaman, O.M. (1992). Fertility decline in Nigeria: the case of Ekpoma Region, Bendel State. *Habitat International.* 16 (1), pp 113-120.

This article identifies some socioeconomic and cultural determinants of fertility and the prospects of its decline in the Ekpoma Region of Nigeria. The findings of the study reveal that for all selected characteristics, the standardised mean births decreased with age. With better education, rising age at marriage, wider acceptability of contraceptives, the evidently harsh economic conditions and the shift by government from the laissez-faire approach to population issues, it is clear that a period of declining fertility has set in. Therefore, discouraging early marriage, increasing the education of girls, availability and knowledge of contraceptives and family limitations, could further the fertility decline.

406. Oheneba-Sakyi, Y. (1989). Cohort Shifts in the Timing of Births in Ghana. *Sociological Perspectives.* Vol. 32, No.4, pp 485-500.

Based on the results of the Ghana Fertility Survey 1979, the author explores the evidence of fertility change based on cohort analysis. He finds evidence of a pattern of lengthened birth interval among the recent cohorts in Ghana, which suggests the influence of spacing behaviour, which might reduce the ultimate family size.

407. Oheneba-Sakyi, Y., K. Awusabo-Asare, E. Gbortsu, A.F. Aryee, (1995). *Female autonomy, decison making, and demographic behaviour among couples in Ghana.* State University of New York (SUNY) Postsdam: Postsdam, New York, University of Ghana, Regional Institute for Population Studies (RIPS), Legon, Ghana. 347 pages.

This study was designed to obtain current information on family relations and demographic behaviour in contemporary Ghana. The fieldwork for the study was carried out in Southern Ghana in 1992. The study sought to find out the relationship, if any between the autonomy of a woman and her interaction with her partner within the context of societal norms, perceptions, and gender roles that shape decisions on family-related issues such as the practice of contraception and ultimate fertility behaviour.

408. Omideyi, A.K. (1993). The emergence of the nuclear family: Its effect on women's roles and fertility change in Nigeria. *Genus,* 49 (1-2): 202-216.

Based on data derived from 2176 married Yoruba women, the author advances the thesis that the emergence of small nuclear family has contributed towards small family sizes among the Yoruba of Nigeria.

409. Omondi-Odhiambo. (1997). Men's Participation in Family Planning Decisions in Kenya. *Population Studies,* 51, pp 29-40.

The study measures the effects of men's participation in family planning decisions, and identifies the conditions, which would stimulate greater participation by men in family planning decisions. The principal conclusions are that Kenyan men do participate in these decisions, take an interest in planning their families, support family planning and use contraception to achieve their goals. The recent transition to lower fertility is probably due, at least in part to changes in men's attitudes.

410. Onuoha, N. (1992). Contributions of the proximate determinants to fertility change in Senegal. *Social Science and Medicine,* vol. 35, no. 10, pp. 1317-1320.

The author examines the contributions of the proximate determinants on fertility change in Senegal using data obtained from the 1978 World Fertility Survey and the 1986 Demographic and Health Survey data. The analysis shows that the magnitude of the change is greatest in contraceptive use, moderate in marriage but least in duration of breastfeeding. The author argues that the impact of the nuptiality index on fertility change lies between contraception and breast-feeding.

411. Onuoha, N. & I.N. Timaeus (1995). Has a fertility transition begun in West Africa? *Journal of international Development.* 7 (1), pp 93-116.

This article examines changing patterns of reproduction in Senegal and Ghana, where both World Fertility Survey and Demographic and Health Surveys have been conducted. It seeks to determine whether a fertility transition has begun in these countries, examining fertility levels and trends, changes in marriage pattern, contraceptive use, breastfeeding, postpartum abstinence and their effect on family building patterns. The study concludes that although a transition to the control of fertility by contraceptive means has begun in both countries, the transition to low fertility is likely to progress slowly.

412. Orubuloye, I. (1995). The demographic situation in Nigeria and prospects for fertility transition. *Journal of International Development.* 7 (1), pp 135-144.

Data sources from the 1980s are used to examine the main features of Nigeria's population patterns and trends. Fertility has remained relatively constant up til very recently, when there has been evidence for a decline in fertility in the south of the country. In the north fertility remains high, contraceptive use remains low, and women continue to marry at young ages.

413. Osei-Hwedie, K. & B. Osei-Hwedie. (1992). Reflections on Zambia's demographic profile and population policy. *Journal of Social Development in Africa.* 7, (10). pp. 87-97.

Zambia's demographic situation is characterised by three dominant features. A high rate of natural increase, massive urbanisation, and wide variations in fertility and mortality levels between the provinces. This paper describes the nature of Zambia's demographic situation, which eventually led to the formulation of a national population policy, the policy instrument and some of the measures necessary for the effective implementation of the policy.

414. Osman, E. A. (1995). *The Fertility Impact of Rural Development Projects: The Case of the Rahad irrigation Project, Sudan*. Ph.D. Dissertation Brown University, 270 pages.

The study examines the impact of the Rahad irrigation and agricultural resettlement project of Central Sudan on fertility behaviour. The findings of the study suggest that program quality was strongly associated with fertility decline.

415. Parr, N.J. (1996). Changes in the factors affecting fertility in Ghana during the early stages of the fertility decline. *Actuarial Studies and Demography Research Paper Series 3,* No. 013-96, Aug 1996. 8 pages. Macquarie University, School of Economics and Financial Studies, Sydney, Australia.

Fertility change in Ghana is examined based on data from GDHS 1988 and GDHS 1993. The main proximate determinant of the decline in fertility is contraception. Other important factors contributing indirectly to the decline are the womans age, education, religion, place of residence and child mortality. The study concludes that the most significant change in Ghanaian fertility has been the decline in fertility in urban areas outside the Greater Accra region.

416. Population Impact Project. (PIP). Department of Geography University of Ghana (1995). Fertility Decline in Ghana 1988-1993. *Population, Environment & Development in Ghana. Population Impact Project* Vol.1 No.1 July 1995.

This issue of PIP's Magazine highlights among other things, Ghana's recent fertility decline and expresses disappointment at the low contraceptive levels in the country. It notes that there is a need to intensify information, education and communication programmes, particularly for expanding the use of family planning.

417. Population Reference Bureau. (PRB). (1993). Is Africa's birth rate falling?

World Population Data Sheet 1993. Population Reference Bureau Washington DC

In a reaction to the initial fertility declines documented in Sub-Saharan Africa, the PRB argues that despite these declines the recent changes do not give the assurance that an imminent change in fertility is taking place in Sub-Saharan Africa.

418. Population Reference Bureau (PRB). (1992). *Africa Demographic and Health Surveys.* Population Reference Bureau.

This book provides information on fertility trends in Sub-Saharan Africa for some selected countries. The data is based on the World Fertility Survey 1977-1982, Contraceptive Prevalence Survey 1984, and Demographic and Health Surveys 1988-1990.

419. Poukouta, P. (1994). The fertility of the Herero of Ngamiland: is there evidence of recent decline? *Population Research Institute Working Paper,* No.94-19, Jul 1994. 38 pages. Pennsylvania State University, Population Research Institute, University Park, Pennsylvania.

The author examines recent trends in fertility among the Herero of rural north western Botswana based on data from a survey carried out by the author in 1993 and other sources. The findings of the study suggest that, in contrast to Botswana as a whole, where fertility has declined, fertility has increased in recent years among the Herero as part of a general strategy to cope with harsh socio-economic conditions caused by drought.

420. Price, N. (1996). The Changing value of children among the Kikuyu of Central Province, Kenya. *Africa,* vol. 66. (3) pp. 411-436.

The study is based on fieldwork undertaken in two ethnically homogenous kikuyu communities, a rural sub location and a peri-urban setting. The study revealed significant variation in the value of children and in fertility motives in the two ethnically homogenous communities.

421. Renne, E. P. (1995). Houses, fertility, and the Nigerian Land Use Act. *Population and Development Review.* 21 (1), pp 113-126.

The study examines the possible implications for fertility decline of changes in the distribution and allocation of family houses and houseplots in a village in South Western Nigeria. Land tenure here traditionally derives from kinship ties, but increasingly, land is being procured by non-family members through cash payments. The Federal Land Use act discourages the sale of rural land, and is often seen as encouraging the need for many children in order to maintain ones property holdings.

The study underscores the importance of political economy in the understanding of fertility change.

422. Renne, E.P. (1996). Shifting boundaries of fertility change in Southwestern Nigeria. *Health Transition Review Supplement* 6, pp 169-190.

The author provides anthropological perspectives towards an understanding of fertility change in South Western Nigeria. This is done by highlighting the changes in social life, family land, marriage, and foster parenthood in the Ekiti area of Southwestern Nigeria.

423. Robinson W. C. (1992). Kenya enters the Fertility transition. *Population Studies* no 46 pp 445-457.

The author examines the recent fertility decline in Kenya and argues that the decline is attributed to rapidly changing attitudes about family size and increasing contraceptive use.

424. Robinson W.C. & Harbison S.F (1995). The Fertility Decline in Kenya. *Journal Of International Development*, 7. pp. 81-92.

This article examines the recent fertility decline in Kenya. The findings of the study show that there has been a rise in contraceptive prevalence and that fertility has fallen. These changes are attributed to the relatively high levels of education, availability of health services, exposure to modernising media and urban lifestyles and a greatly strengthened family planning service delivery system.

425. Rutenberg, N. (1995). *Fertility Change in Ghana: Findings from the 1993 DHS.* Options Project USAID Contract No. DPE-3035-Q-00-0054-00. 25 pages.

The study looks at the evidence of the recent fertility decline in Ghana based on the 1993 Demographic and Health Survey. Three main questions are addressed in the report. Is the fertility decline reported in the DHS valid and correct? Second, what is a responsible estimate of contraceptive prevalence and what has been the impact of contraceptive use on fertility? Third, are there important factors in addition to contraceptive use that have contributed to the decline in fertility? The study argues that the results of the DHS on fertility and contraceptive practice appear plausible and it is likely that this demand will persist into the near future.

426. Safilios-Rothschild, C. (1988). *Women's Income profile as a key indicator of the status of women for the understanding of changing fertility behaviour.* Paper presented at the conference on women's position and demographic change in the course of development, Asker (Oslo), 15-18 June, 1988.

The study examines the characteristics of women's income in two rural communities in Kenya and the relative importance of women's education and women's income profile for women's fertility behaviour as well as for the proximate determinants of fertility. The villages were selected so as to represent not only different ethnic groups but also different levels of socio-economic development and a different status of women. The analysis of the data shows that women's income is significantly related to children-specific expenses undertaken by women. The higher the woman's income, the more they spend for children, that is for children's clothes and school fees. The finding indicates that when women's income is substantial (within the context of rural Kenya), women's aspirations for their children increase and they are willing to invest more money to realise these aspirations. Under these conditions, children become costly to mothers and mothers' demand for children is diminished since they no longer rely solely on their children for labour.

427. Scriber, S. (1995). Policies affecting fertility and contraceptive use: an assessment of twelve Sub-Saharan African countries. *World Bank Discussion Papers 259,* 81.

The report identifies Botswana, Zimbabwe and Kenya as countries that have population policies most conducive to fertility decline. Countries such as Mali, Uganda, Cote d'Ivoire have policies that are least conducive to fertility decline, whereas countries such as Burundi, Ghana, Nigeria, Senegal, Tanzania and Togo fall between the two extremes.

428. Shapiro, D. & B.O. Tambashe. (1994). Education, employment and fertility in Kinshasa and prospects for changes in reproductive behaviour. *Population Research Institute Working Paper, No.* 1994-06, Jan 1994, 26 (8) pages. Pennsylvania State University, University Park, Pennsylvania.

Data from a 1990 survey of some 2400 women of reproductive age in Kinshasa, Zaire are used to examine the relationships linking women's education, employment, and fertility behaviour. The findings of the study show that modern contraception and abortion are alternative fertility control strategies in Kinshasa, with abortion appearing to play an important role in contributing to the observed fertility differentials by education and employment.

429. Shapiro, D. (1996). Fertility Decline in Kinshasa. *Population Studies.* 50 (1), pp. 89-103.

This paper examines key socio-economic changes over the past 40 years in the lives of women in Kinshasa, Zaire and how these changes relate to observe fertility behaviour. Data from surveys carried out in 1955, 1975 and 1990 are used to highlight the remarkable shift that has taken place in the educational attainment of women. In the 1950s the vast majority of adult women had no formal education, while by 1990 the median woman had been to secondary school. This dramatic shift was accompanied by several related changes, including delays in age at marriage and increased participation in the labour market. Total fertility, which was estimated at 7.5 in the 1950s and had not changed much by 1975, appears to have fallen more recently, by about 1.5 children or more. The decline in fertility appears to be closely linked to the improvements in secondary schooling for women in Kinshasa.

430. Sokari-George, E., Emeruem, J.O, Dimpa-Harry S. H. (1991). Rural electrification: a study of socio-economic and fertility change in Rivers State, Nigeria. *African Study Monographs,* Vol. 12, No.4, Dec 1991. pp 167-83. Kyoto, Japan.

The impact of rural electrification on fertility change was examined in Rivers State in Nigeria. The focus was on two areas, one with electricity and the other without electricity. The findings of the study revealed that family planning was more practised in the electrified community than the non-electrified one. The implications are that rural electrification could contribute to fertility decline.

431. Statistical Service of Ghana (1994). *Ghana Demographic and Health Survey 1993.* Columbia, MD. Institute for Resource Development.

This survey is the second demographic survey undertaken in the country under the auspices of the Statistical Service of Ghana and Macro International Institute. The findings of the survey lend support to a decline in fertility compared to the previous survey conducted in 1988.

432. Takyi, B.A. & Y. Oheneba-Sakyi. (1994). Customs, Practices, Family Life, and Marriage in Contemporary Ghana, West Africa. *Family Perspective,* 28, (4): pp 257-281.

The study looks at contemporary changes in family life in Ghana. It reports on the trends in fertility, the structure of the Ghanaian family, and the circumstances that are part of the family formation processes and subsequent fertility related patterns in contemporary Ghana. The study links the changes primarily to economic and social forces.

433. Tambashe, B. O & D. Shapiro. (1996). Family background and early life course transitions in Kinshasa. *Journal of Marriage and the Family,* Vol. 58, No.4 pp 1029-37. Minneapolis, Minnesota.

The study examines the influence of some aspects of women's family background on transitions to sexual activity, marriage and motherhood. The study is based on a sample of approximately 2400 women aged 13-49 surveyed in Kinshasa, Zaire in

1990. The results of the study suggest that continued increases in educational levels should contribute to delays in these life-course transitions and ultimately to some reductions in fertility.

434. Tanzania Bureau of Statistics; Macro International. Demographic and Health Surveys (DHS) (Calverton, Maryland). *Tanzania Demographic and Health Survey,* 1996. Aug 1997. 312 pages. Dares Salaam, Tanzania. (1997).

This book summarises the findings of the 1996 Tanzania DHS, a nationally representative survey of 8,120 women aged 15-49 and 2,256 men aged 15-59. The study summarises basic information on fertility, mortality and other issues. It provides evidence of a significant decline in fertility in Tanzania.

435. Tawiah, E.O. (1997). Factors affecting contraceptive use in Ghana. *Journal of Biosocial Science,* Vol. 29. pp 141-149.

The author examines factors that affect the use of contraception in Ghana based on data derived from the 1988 Ghana Demographic and Health Survey. The findings of the study reveal that the relatively low fertility of women with higher education is largely attributable to a high level of contraceptive use. The findings suggest that a certain education threshold is necessary for women to use contraception.

436. Thomas, D. & I. Muvandi. (1994). The Demographic transition in Southern Africa: Reviewing the evidence from Botswana and Zimbabwe. *Demography,* vol. 31 no 2 p 217-227.

The study examines the onset of fertility transition in Botswana and Zimbabwe based on a comparision of the 1984 CPS and the 1988 DHS. The authors argue that part, not all, of the observed decline in the number of children ever born reported in the 1984 CPS and the 1988 DHS in Botswana and Zimbabwe can be attributed to differences in sample composition. Women in the 1988 survey appear to be better educated than women of the same cohort in the 1984 survey. Blanc and Rustein argue that differences in education levels in the pairs of surveys are not significant. They also claim that these differences do not account for any of the observed decline in fertility between the surveys of women aged 15 to 49. The authors stand by their conclusions and argue for caution when aggregate statistics from the CPS and the DHS are used to make projections about the course of fertility and population growth in Botswana and Zimbabwe.

437. Thomas, D. & I. Muvandi. (1994). How fast is fertility declining in Botswana and Zimbabwe? *World Bank Discussion Paper,* 258. 31pp.

It has been argued that Botswana and Zimbabwe are on the path of the demographic transition in Sub-Saharan Africa. The data base for this assertion comes from the contraceptive Prevalence Surveys (CPS) and Demographic Health Survey (DHS) which were conducted in both countries. This paper examines the comparability of these data sources and finds that at least part of the observed decline in aggregate fertility rates in both countries can be attributed to differences in sample composition. The study concludes that there is evidence that differences in the structure of the instruments also raise questions about the comparability of the two data sources.

438. Udjo, E.O. (1991). Fertility levels among Nigeria's Kanuri. *Genus,* vol. 47, pp 163-76.

This article analyses and evaluates information from maternity histories collected from retrospective survey carried out by the author in some parts of Northern Nigeria, which would supplement our meagre knowledge of levels and patterns of fertility in Northern Nigeria. Estimates of total fertility rates appear plausible but low by African standards. This low fertility is attributable to sterility. There is no direct evidence as to the cause of the sterility but fragmentary evidence points to prevalence of venereal disease in the area.

439. Udjo, E.O. (1996). Is fertility falling in Zimbabwe? *Journal of Biosocial Science,* 28 (1): 25-35.

The author examines the recent fertility decline in Zimbabwe against the background of the country's relatively high contraceptive prevalence rate of 43 percent among currently married women. The study uses data from several surveys in Zimbabwe, especially birth histories of the Zimbabwe DHS. The findings of the study reveal that the fertility decline in Zimbabwe is modest and that the decline is concentrated among high order births. Multivariate analysis did not show a statistically significant effect of contraception on fertility, partly because a high proportion of Zimbabwean women in the reproductive age groups never use contraception due to prevailing pronatalist attitudes in the country.

440. Uitto, J. I. (1992). Fertility transition and socio-economic change in western Kenya. *African Study Monographs,* Vol. 13, No. 4, Dec 1992. 185-201 pp. Kyoto, Japan.

Differences in fertility between the various regions of Kenya are analysed and explained. Different stages of the fertility transition are observed in the different regions of Kenya depending on the particular socio-economic situation, but these differences are likely to even out in the future.

441. United Nations, Economic Commission for Africa (ECA) (Addis Ababa, Ethiopia). (1992). *Strategies to improve contraceptive use to influence demographic*

trends in African countries. No. ECA|POP|TP|92|1(2b), Dec 1992. VI, 49 pp. Addis Ababa, Ethiopia.

This report describes current levels of contraceptive knowledge and usage in Africa and examines strategies for future improvement. A review of the contraceptive methods most widely used and of the impact of contraceptive use on demographic trends is discussed.

442. Vanderpost, C. (1992). Regional patterns of fertility transition in Botswana. *Geography,* Vol. 77, pp. 102-122.

The author examines regional patterns of fertility transition in Botswana. He argues that the fertility transition in Botswana is progressing in a geographically uneven manner. In some districts fertility is increasing due to breakdown of traditions, while in others it is slowly declining due to modernisation or westernisation. He stresses the importance of diffusion in accounting for the observed patterns in fertility in Botswana.

443. Van de Walle, E. & A. Foster. (1990). *Fertility decline in Africa: assessment and prospects. World Bank Technical Paper, 125,* (Africa Technical Department Series):

The study is among the first reactions to Africa's fertility transition. Based on their assessment of the decline, the authors express doubt as to whether Sub-Saharan Africa is really on course in the fertility transition.

444. Ware, H. (1994). Thoughts on the course of fertility transition in Sub-Saharan Africa. In T. Locoh & V. Hetrich (eds.). *The Onset of fertility transition in Sub-Saharan Africa.* International Union for the Scientific Study of Population. pp 199-296.

The author provides some thoughts on the recent fertility decline in Sub-Saharan Africa. She argues among other things that it would have been reassuring if an independent study other than Demographic and Health Surveys data were conducted for each country in order to enhance our understanding of the emerging fertility trends in Sub-Saharan Africa.

445. Westoff, C. (1992). Age at first marriage, age at first birth, and fertility in Africa. *World Bank Technical Paper,* 169, 57 pages.

This study examines trends in marriage and age at first birth in some African countries based on the findings of the World Fertility Survey and the Demographic and Health Surveys. A pattern of rapidly increasing age at marriage and first birth is shown for some countries, while others exhibit the beginnings of such change. The paper explains the demographic significance of such changes, and a model of fertility is constructed. It is suggested that population policies aimed at reducing fertility should include efforts to encourage the postponement of the first birth by raising the age at marriage.

446. Westoff, C. & G. Rodriguez. (1993). The Mass Media and Family Planning in Kenya. *DHS Working Paper No 4.* Columbia, MD. Macro International.

The study looks at the effects of mass media on family planning in Kenya. It looks at the possibilities and essential problems in mass media effects on family planning in Kenya.

447. Westoff, C. & A. Bankole. (1997). Mass media and reproductive behaviour in Africa. *DHS Analytical Report, No.2,* April 1997. 39 pages. *Macro International, Demographic and Health Surveys (DHS),* Calverton, Maryland.

The study examines the contribution of modern mass media to fertility reduction in societies with traditional notions of early childbearing and large families. The data are derived from DHS surveys in Burkina Faso, Ghana, Kenya, Madagascar, Namibia, and Zambia, and from similar survey carried out in Morocco. The general conclusion drawn from the study is that there is a persistent and frequently strong association between exposure to mass media and reproductive behaviour in Africa in the expected direction, and that such exposure is directly related to greater knowledge and use of contraception, intention to use contraception in the future, preferences for fewer children, and intention to stop childbearing. In addition, there is evidence that media exposure is also associated with later age at marriage. These conclusions are generalizable to women and men, both married and single.

448. Wortham, R. (1993). Population growth and the demographic transition in Kenya. *International Sociology,* 8: pp 197-214.

This paper focuses on patterns of population growth in Kenya. The historical pattern of population growth from the close of the 19th century to 1992 is explored in the first two major sections. The applicability of demographic transition theory to the study of population growth and development in Kenya is addressed in the third section. Kenya is observed to have passed through the underdeveloped stage characterised by increasing birth and death rates and entered the transition stage during the 1980s. Issues concerning the prospects of substantial continued reductions in the fertility level are addressed in the concluding section.

449. Wortham, R. (1995). Prospects for fertility reduction and projections for future population growth in Kenya. *Population Research and Policy Review,* 14

(1), pp 111-135.

Prospects for fertility reduction and projection for future population growth in Kenya are analysed. Four population projections are discussed. Each of these projections assume that there will be fertility reduction. It is suggested that Kenya will probably not complete the demographic transition before the year 2050, but Kenya should continue to move through the transition stage.

450. Yamuah, M. (1993). Population growth in the Gambia and Swaziland. In *International Population Conference: Montreal 1993, Volume 2. 1993.* 345-52 pp. International Union for the Scientific Study of Population (IUSSP), Liege, Belgium.

The author investigates recent changes in fertility, mortality and international migration in the Gambia and Swaziland, with a focus on the implications for future population growth.

5

Fertility Decline in Developing Countries: General Literature

451. Althaus, S.F. (1991). Early Marriage and Childbearing Remain Common in much of the Developing World Even as Fertility Falls. *International Family Planning Perspectives* Vol. 17, No 3 Sept pp 119-120.

The author examines levels and trends in fertility in some developing countries, and observes that childbearing still begins early in much of the developing World though fertility is falling.

452. Bahr, J. & P. Gans. (1991). Regional fertility differentials in developing countries. *Kieler-Geographische-Schriften,* 78, pp 313-337.

The author's advance the thesis that if we wish to explain observed fertility differences satisfactorily we must incorporate regional factors that go beyond socio-economic and demographic differentials within a population more than has been done so far.

453. Bongaarts, J. (1986). Contraceptive use and annual acceptors required for fertility transition. Results of a projection model. *Studies in Family Planning,* 17 (5) pp 209-16.

Fertility declines in developing countries are usually accompanied by large increases in contraceptive use and in the number of new acceptors. Based on a target setting model, this article makes hypothetical projections to estimate prevalence in contraceptive use and number of new acceptors over the course of the fertility transition. It concludes that to attain replacement level of fertility, a contraceptive usage rate of about 75 percent is needed. Trends in new acceptors are found to be very sensitive to discontinuation rate changes, and it is thus generally difficult to estimate fertility trends by examining trends in numbers of acceptors.

454. Bongaarts, J. (1995). The role of family planning programs in contemporary fertility transitions. *Population Council Research Division Working Paper,* vol. 71, 31 pp. Population Council, Research Division. New York.

The implementation of family planning programs has been the principal population policy instrument in the developing world in the past few decades. This paper reviews the controversy over the role these programs have played in reducing fertility. Opposing views in a number of contentious issues for example the significance of unmet need and unwanted fertility is summarised and a consensus position is presented.

455. Bongaarts, J. (1993). The Fertility Impact of Family Planning Programs. *Research Division Population Council Working Papers 1993 no 47,* 35 pages.

This study provides new estimates of both the gross and net impact of family planning programs. Gross measures are easier to calculate, but they do not take into account the potentially significant substitution and catalytic effects of programs. These factors are incorporated in net measures, which are therefore preferable for most policy purposes. The average net program impact in the developing world in the late 1980s is estimated at 1.4 births per woman. This implies that organised family planning programs have been responsible for about half of the fertility decline that has occurred since the 1950s.

456. Cleland, J. & J. Hobcraft. (Eds.) (1985). *Reproductive Change in Developing Countries. Insights from the World Fertility Survey.* Oxford University Press. 295 pages.

The book is concerned with reviewing results from the WFS and assessing their consequences for demographic knowledge of the Third World. The book is divided into twelve chapters and covers several aspects of reproduction in developing countries.

457. Cleland, J. (1996). A Regional Review of Fertility Trends in Developing Countries: 1960-1990 In *The Future Population of the World: What Can We Assume Today?* pp 47-72 Edited by Wolfgang Lutz. Revised Edition.

This study provides a review of fertility trends in developing countries over the period 1960 to 1995. It adopts a regional perspective comprising of East and Southeast Asia, South Asia, Latin America, the Arab States, and Sub-Saharan Africa.

458. Coale, A. (1983). Recent Trends in Fertility in Less Developed Countries. *Science,* Vol. 221, pp 829-832.

The rate of increase of population in less developed countries accelerated rapidly from 1850 to 1960 because of a rapid decline in mortality while fertility remained high. In the 1960's, the birth rate as a whole began to decline more rapidly than the death rate-very rapidly in some populations, most notably in China. The study concludes that the momentum of growth implies continued increase in populations for several decades even in countries where fertility has fallen the most and very large additional increases where there has been no decline in the rate of childbearing.

459. Demeny, P. (1990). Global population trends. *Environmental Impact Assessment Review,* 10 (4) pp 323-334.

Analysis of the latest statistics for global population growth, with an estimated global total of 8 billion by 2020 is made. Special attention is given to world mortality and fertility trends. The study proposes that fertility in the developing world will decline below 3.5 children per mother by 2000 for most countries except Africa.

460. Donaldson, P.J & A. O. Tsui. (1990). The International Family Planning Movement. *Population Bulletin,* 45, 3, 46 pages.

The number of women using family planning has increased six fold to over 400 million married women of childbearing age within the past three decades. The study argues that the evolution of behaviour and attitudes toward using birth control among Third World couples reflects the goals and hard work of an international network of individuals, governments and organisations. Among the world regions, contraceptive use ranges from about 17 percent in Africa to 75 percent in Asia. In some African countries, however, family planning is still a foreign concept, and fewer than 5 percent of women use any birth control. The study concludes that world wide increase in the practice of family planning has led to fertility declines in many Third World countries, slowing rapid population growth rates.

461. Egero, B. & M. Hammarskjold. (1994). *Understanding reproductive change: Kenya, Tamil Nadu, and Punjab, Costa Rica.* 1994 167 pages. Lund University press Lund. Sweden. Chartwell Bratt, Bromley, England.

This collection of four case studies examines the reasons for the trend toward lower fertility in developing countries. The focus is on identifying the forces that motivate people living under different conditions to reduce the size of their families. Kenya is one of the few countries in Sub-Saharan Africa displaying a distinct trend to lower fertility. In India, Tamil Nadu and Punjab are widely different in socio-economic development, yet both have seen significant reductions in fertility. In Costa Rica, a stable trend of fertility decline was halted with the economic stagnation around 1980, only to resume in recent years. In the introductory chapter, the country studies are analysed against current understanding of the demographic transition as it took place in Europe, and the more recent processes in East and South-east Asia.

462. El-Badry, M.A. (1992). World Population Change: a long- range perspective. *Ambio,* 21 (1) pp 18-23.

Analysis of the world population change is made. Measures such as fertility, mortality and age-structure are analysed from the middle of the 20th century and extending through the 21st century. The data is drawn from the estimates and projections prepared by the UN Population Division.

463. Freedman, R. & A.K. Blanc. (1992). Fertility Transition. An Update. *International Family Planning Perspectives.* Vol. 18 no 2.

The study looks at fertility trends in developing countries based on United Nations data. It is observed that fertility in the developing world declined by almost one-third between the period 1965-1970. Different patterns of the transition are observed for Latin America, Asia and Africa. It is argued that as fertility has decreased, declines have also occurred in the number of years between a woman's first birth and her last birth and in the number of years the average woman spends caring for small children.

464. Hill, K. (1992). Fertility and mortality trends in the developing world. *Ambio,* 21, 1 pp 79-83.

Fertility and mortality have declined substantially in the developing world over the last 30 years. The pace of the decline in mortality has been fairly constant across regions, but the pace of decline in fertility has varied widely, having been fastest in East and Southeast Asia and slowest in Africa. With both fertility and mortality declining, the growth rate of the population of the developing world has remained approximately constant at around 2 percent per annum over the last 30 years. Both fertility and mortality are expected to continue to decline in the foreseeable future, but the growth rate is also expected to decline to about 1.2 per annum by 2000.

465. Horiuchi, S. (1992). Stagnation in the decline of the world population growth rate during the 1980s. *Science,* 257 (5071), pp 761-765.

The World population growth rate has gone through three phases in the second part of the 20th century. These were a rise in the 1950s and 1960s caused by the global decline in death rates and a fall in the 1970s brought about mainly by the reduction of fertility in a number of developing countries. The stagnation of growth rate decline in the 1980s could be attributed to three main factors; the decline in fertility around 1970 and a stall in this decline around 1980 in both India and China; a change in the age structure of population in favour of higher birth rates, and thirdly, the fact that few developing countries have started fertility declines since the declines in the early 1970s. There has thus been a deepening of the gap in fertility levels between developed and developing countries.

466. Iverson, S.B. (1992). *Evolutionary demographic transition theory: comparative causes of prehistoric, historic and modern demographic transitions.* PhD dissertation, University of Florida 149 pages.

A general theory of the demographic transition is developed based on the experiences of Barbados, Kuwait, Mauritius, and Zimbabwe. The study concludes that changes in reproductive behaviour are an adaptive response to changing material conditions, and that the most important factors associated with modern fertility declines are economic or unemployment conditions that conflict with reproduction and women's access to material resources independent of men and children.

467. Keyfitz, N. (1992). Completing the world wide demographic transition. The relevance of past experience. *Ambio,* 21 (1), pp 26-30.

In looking at the world population problem, the author argues that if there is one universal human right it is the right to limit the number of ones offspring. Besides this, it is also argued that the application of this principle may not solve the entire population problem, but it will deal with a considerable part of it.

468. Kocher, J.E. (1972). Rural socio-economic stratification and fertility decline in developing countries. *East African Universities. Social Science Conference. Annual Conference,* 1972, Nairobi.

The author looks at the influence of rural socio-economic stratification on fertility decline in developing countries.

469. Kono, S. & H. Yasuko. (1994). Fertility in the developing countries: a comparative study of the Demographic and Health Surveys. *IDS Statistical Data Series,* No. 66, 1994. 310 pages. Institute of Developing Economics (IDE), Tokyo, Japan.

An analysis of fertility differentials and the determinants of population growth in developing countries are presented, based on data from 28 countries that took part in Phase I of the Demographic and Health Surveys Program. This volume focused on comparative studies on the levels and trends of fertility, proximate determinants of fertility, socio-economic determinants and reproductive behaviour. Case studies are included on Bangladesh, Indonesia, Japan, Sri Lanka, Taiwan, and Thailand, and on the effects of mass media on contraception and fertility in Africa.

470. Kono, S. & Y. Hayase. (Eds.) (1994). *Fertility in the developing countries. A Comparative study of the Demographic and Health Surveys*. IDE Statistical Data Series No. 66. Institute of Developing Economies, Tokyo, Japan. 1994. 310 pages.

The study examines fertility differential and the main causes of the population growth in less developed countries mainly based on data in 28 developing countries. The present volume focused on comparative studies on the levels and trends of fertility, proximate determinants of fertility, socio-economic determinants and reproductive behaviour in the less developed countries. The report analyses the conditions of fertility decline by using different analytical techniques and viewpoints.

471. Kono, S. (1994). A Comparative study of fertility levels and trends in developing countries. In S. Kono and Y. Hayashe (eds.) (1994). *Fertility in the developing countries. A Comparative study of the Demographic and Health Surveys*. IDE Statistical data Deries No. 66. Institute of Developing Economies Tokyo, Japan, 1994, pp 7-28.

The study presents a review of the current levels and trends in fertility in developing countries and provides some of the state of the art pertaining to the recent theories and hypotheses on determinants of fertility changes therein. The study argues that inspite of the diversities and heterogeneity of the developing world, a strong statement can be made that fertility has been declining one by one, some being faster and in a wider step and the other slower and to a lesser extent, trailing the paths that European countries experienced in the 19th and sometimes in the early 20th century.

472. Lee, B. S. & G. P. Louis. (1993). The influence of rural-urban migration on migrants fertility in Korea, Mexico and Cameroon. *Population Research and Policy Review*, Vol. 12, No.1, 1993, pp 3-26. Dordrecht, Netherlands.

This paper presents a comparative analysis of the relationship between rural-urban migration and fertility in South Korea, Mexico, and Cameroon. Using an autoregressive model, the results show a significant rural-urban migration adaptation effect in Korea and Mexico, a reduction of 2.57 and 1.45 children during the entire childbearing period, respectively, when compared to a rural stayer, even after the effect of selection has been controlled. Rural-urban migration has a very small impact on fertility in Cameroon due to the fact that the fertility-increasing effect of urban residency on the improve supply conditions of births, such as reduced infertility, offsets the fertility-depressing effect of urban residency on the demand for births.

473. Mason, A. (1993). The response of fertility and mortality to economic crisis and structural adjustment policy during the 1980s: A review. In *International Population Conference Montreal 1993*, Vol. 2, 1993, pp 411-29. International Union for the Scientific Study of Population (IUSSP), Liege, Belgium.

The purpose of this paper is to review the demographic experience of the 1980s and to assess the impact of economic crisis. Two main conclusions are drawn. The first is that structural adjustment policies have had adverse and unanticipated effects on mortality or fertility undermining important social objectives of development. A second possibility is that mortality has increased or fertility decline has slowed because of economic problems, which are unrelated to structural adjustment policies. The geographical focus is on developing countries.

474. Mauldin W. P. & J. A. Ross. (1994). Prospects and programs for fertility reduction, 1990-2015. *Studies in Family Planning,* 25, pp 77-95.

This article examines the likelihood that each of the 37 developing countries with populations of 15 million or more in 1990 will reach replacement fertility by the year 2015? For this article, a composite index was used as the basis for predicting future levels of total fertility. The index was constructed from socio-economic variables, total fertility rates for the years 1985-90, total fertility rate decline from 1960-65 to 1985-90, family planning program effort scores in 1989, and the level of contraceptive prevalence in 1990. Eight countries are classified, as certain to reach replacement fertility by 2015 and an additional thirteen probably will also. Five countries are classified as possibly reaching replacement fertility, and eleven as unlikely to do so.

475. McHenry, J.P. (1991). *Socio-economic development and fertility decline: an application of the Easterlin Synthesis approach to data from the World Fertility Survey. Colombia, Costa Rica, Sri Lanka and Tunisia.* UN Department of International Economic and Social Affairs, New York, New York. 115 pages.

This study is part of a project investigating the relationship between socio-economic factors and fertility decline in developing countries through a comparative analysis involving five country case studies. Four of those countries are included here: Colombia, Costa Rica, Sri Lanka and Tunisia and data are from the WFS. The results suggest that if the dominant effect of marriage duration is interpreted primarily as a control variable for exposure to intercourse, contraceptive usage and secondary sterility are the major remaining intermediate variables affecting fertility. They also indicate that with regard to the Easterlin- Crimmins empirical formulation of contraceptive motivation, although the theoretical concept is a promising one, more empirical and statistical attention is required so as to improve the estimator.

476. McNicoll, G. (1991). Changing fertility patterns and fertility policies in the third world. *Working Papers in Demography. Australian National University, Research School of Social Sciences, Division of Demography and Sociology, Canberra, Australia.* No.32, 1991 37 pages.

The study examines fertility changes and policies in developing countries. Some of the items discussed in the publication include data collection, regional fertility patterns, explanations and interpretations, and an assessment of fertility policies.

477. Muhuri, P.K, A.K. Blanc, S.O. Rustein. (1994). Socio-economic differentials in fertility. *DHS Comparative Studies, No. 13,* May, 79 pages. Macro International, Demographic and Health Surveys, Calverton, Maryland.

Socio-economic differentials in fertility in 33 countries that took part in Demographic and Health Surveys conducted in the late 1980s and early 1990s are provided. After a description of the methodology, measures of fertility are provided based on the education of the woman, her current work status, place of residence, migration status and the occupation and education of the husband. The study also provides trends in socio-economic differentials in fertility for 21 countries for which data are available from both the World Fertility Survey (WFS) and DHS.

478. Ofosu, Y. (1994). Policies and fertility transitions in the third world: failures, successes, and uncertainties. *World Employment Programme Working paper: Labour and Population,* No.189, 40 pages.

Reasons why fertility has declined so significantly throughout the developing world, including Sub-Saharan Africa where the decline has not been so dramatic, are explored.

479. Phillips, D. (1994). Epidemiological transition: Implications for health and health care provision. *Geografiska Annaler,* 76B, pp 71-89.

The article discusses the general concept of epidemiological transition and its manifestations in three case studies drawn from Hong Kong, Thailand and Mauritius. Birth rates changes over time are provided in order to see the linkages between epidemiological changes and demographic outcomes.

480. Population Division of the Department of International Economic and Social Affairs, United Nations Secretariat (1987). World Demographic Trends. *World Health Statistics Quarterly,* 40 (1), pp. 6-21.

The study provides an overview of world demographic trends. It is shown that the world population doubled over the period 1950 to 1985. This is attributed to the significant decline in fertility recorded in many countries in Latin America and Asia during the period centred around 1970.The study shows that significant fertility decline has not started in the majority of countries in Africa, and mortality, although still very high, is declining particularly for infants and children, resulting in very high growth rates and increasingly younger age structures. The situation is completely different from the developed countries, which are characterised by low rates of population growth, low levels of fertility and mortality, and an increasing proportion of older persons. It is observed that a number of countries have below replacement fertility levels and are projected to reach zero or negative population growth in the near future. If such trends continue there will be a reduction in the proportion of the world population living in the developed regions from one-third in 1950 to one-sixth in 2025.

481. Repetto, R. (1979). *Economic Equality and Fertility in Developing Countries.* Baltimore, John Hopkins University Press 186 pages.

Does a more equal distribution of income lead to lower fertility. The question is conceptually hard to pin down and statistically difficult to answer. The author presents a sophisticated econometric analysis of the income distribution-fertility behaviour relationships across countries and in two specific settings, Puerto Rico and South Korea. His conclusion in each case is that the link exists and warrants a causal interpretation.

482. Riley, N.E. (1997). Gender, Power and Population Change. *Population Bulletin,* Vol. 52, no 1, 48 pages.

The Bulletin explores what gender is, how it is expressed in different societies, and how its various expressions relate to demographic processes. It uses case studies along with more traditional demographic data to explore the complex relationships among gender, power, and population change in non industrialised countries. It also examines how population policies can enhance or retard progress toward greater equality for women.

483. Robey, B., S.O. Rustein, L. Morris. (1993). The fertility decline in developing countries. *Scientific American,* Vol.269, No.6, Dec 1993. pp 60-7. New York, New York.

A general review of recent fertility declines and their causes in developing countries are presented. Data are from a variety of published sources including Demographic and health Surveys. The author's note that, in contrast to the demographic transition undergone by the now developed world, birth rates in the developing world have fallen even in the absence of improved living conditions. The decrease has also proceeded with remarkable speed. Developing countries appear to have benefited from the growing influence and scope of family-planning programs, and from new contraceptive technologies and from the educational power of the mass media.

484. Robey, B. (1993). The birth rate decline in developing countries. *Outlook on Agriculture,* 22 (4) pp 221-224.

This article examines the decline in birth rates in developing countries. It is observed that in the mid-1960s women in Asia, Africa and Latin America gave birth to an average of six children. Today, the average is about four-a drop of one-third. In some regions and countries the average is substantially lower, approaching levels in the developed world. It is something of a surprise to learn that birth rates have declined so rapidly in so many countries, including some that experts considered too poor and traditional for this to occur. Demographic and Health Surveys (DHS) and similar family planning surveys conducted in more than 40 developing countries since 1985 tell the story of this striking decline.

485. Ross, J.A. & W.P. Mauldin. (1996). Family Planning Programs: Efforts and Results, 1972-1994. *Studies in Family Planning,* vol. 27, no 3. pp 137-147.

This study assesses the strength of key elements of national family planning programs for most developing countries for 1972, 1982, 1989, and 1994. Overall program effort for the developing world increased sharply from 1972 to 1982, and again from 1982 to 1989, but only modestly thereafter.

486. Ross, J. A. & W.P. Mauldin. (1994). Effort and achievement in national family planning programmes. *World Health Forum,* 15 (3) pp 251-257.

New data show that national family planning programmes have made impressive progress in the last 25 years. Fertility rates have been reduced dramatically, but during the current decade even greater achievements will be called for. No family planning programme has stopped or reversed growth; the strongest ones have only attenuated it. The age structure of the present population means that, even with the two-child family, births will exceed depths for two or three generations to come, and the worlds population will grow by well over half (58 percent) adding another 3100 million people for a minimum of 8300 million.

487. Singh, R. (1994). *Family planning success stories: Asia, Latin America, and Africa.* 302 pp. UBS Publishers Distributors, New Delhi, India.

The author describes the development of successful policies designed to slow the rate of population growth in a selected number of developing countries around the world. The countries analysed are Thailand, Indonesia, Sri Lanka, Brazil, Colombia, Mexico, Zimbabwe and Tunisia. The emphasis is on the development of successful family planning programs that do not rely on coercive measures to reduce fertility.

488. Teitelbaum, M. (1975). Relevance of the demographic transition theory for developing countries. *Science,* 188 vol. 2. pp. 420-25.

The relevance of the classic demographic transition theory to the developing world is discussed. Comparisons are also made with regards to the European experience.

489. Uitto, J. (1992). Fertility transition and socio-economic change in the developing world: Overview and assessment of interlinkages. *Svensk geografisk årsbok,* 68 pp. 156-169.

The author explores the linkages between fertility transition and socio-economic change in developing countries. He concludes that there exists a clear linkage between poverty and fertility i.e. socio-economic status affects the fertility behaviour of the people. This factor is visible both at family and local levels as well as on macro or global scales.

490. Watkins, S. (1987). The fertility transition: Europe and the third World compared. *Sociological Forum,* vol. 2 no 4, pp. 645-673.

This article is a comparative analysis of the fertility decline in Europe and the Third World. In general, lower levels of fertility have largely been due to the adoption of innovative behaviour, particularly within marriage. Socioeconomic development has been identified as being responsible for fertility differences between groups during the transition, although ideational or institutional change should not be ruled out. The pace and scope of the declines also suggest the involvement of diffusion.

491. Westoff, C., L. Moreno, & N. Goldman. (1989). The Demographic impact of changes in contraceptive practice in Third World Populations. *Population and Development Review,* 15 (1) pp 91-106.

Two questions are posed in this article. The first is how much would fertility decline if unwanted births were prevented? And the second, how much would unwanted fertility decline if contraceptive practice improved? Data collected from eight developing countries in the demographic and health surveys suggest that unless wanted fertility declines further, the opportunity to reduce total fertility would be largely limited. Even in a country like Peru, where a third of births are reported unwanted, the potential for reducing total fertility by increasing effective contraceptive use is very limited.

Author Index

(Based on Entry Numbers in the Text)

Aase, A, 289
Adamchak, D.J, 283-285
Adansi-Pipim, G, 357
Adeokun, L.A, 347
Adepoju, A, 345, 390
Adlakha, A.L, 140, 208
Adomako Ampofo, 337
Aghajanian, A, 141, 254
Agyei-Mensah, S, 286-289
Ainsworth, M, 290
Alan, I, 231
Alba, F, 055
Althaus, S.F, 451
Amin, S, 162-163
Amin, R, 142
Anarfi, J, 291
Ankomah, A, 280
ANON, 143, 144
Aramburu, C, 056, 068
Archer, L, 340-341
Aryee, A.F, 407
Ascadi, G.T.F, 292
Ascadi, J. G, 292
Assogba, L, 357
Atkin, L.C, 071
Awusabo-Asare, K, 407
Axelrod, P, 145
Axinn, W.G, 146-149

Backhaus, T, 150
Bahr, J, 452
Balasubramanian, K, 151
Banister, J, 140
Bankole, A, 293-295, 447
Barbieri, M, 296
Barney, C, 297
Barroso, C, 057
Basu, A.M, 212
Bauni, K, 298
Becker, G.S, 001-002
Belden, P.B, 150
Benefo, K.D, 299
Benneh, G, 300
Berquo, E, 100
Betrand, J.T.E, 298
Bilsborrow, R.E, 124, 169
Blacker, J, 301
Blake, J, 003
Blanc, A.K, 302, 463, 477
Blangero, J, 256
Bongaarts, J, 004-005, 348, 453-455
Bose, A, 152
Boserup, E, 006
Bradley, C, 303-304

Brass, W, 305-306
Bravo, J.H, 058
Brems, S.K, 059
Brockerhoff, M, 307-308
Brown, G.F, 309
Brunborg, H, 310
Bulatao, R.A, 292
Buor, D, 311

Cain, M, 007, 153
Caldwell, B, 154
Caldwell, J.C, 008-010, 155, 156, 297, 312-319
Caldwell, P, 156, 314-318
Campbell, B.O, 157
Campbell, E, 320-321
Campbell, P.G, 320
Carlson, G, 012
Carter, A.T, 011
Carvalho, J.A, 060-062
Casterline, J.B, 013, 040, 048, 120, 158, 243
Chackiel, J, 063
Chakraborty, J, 252
Chamratithirong, A, 194, 201-202, 225
Chang, M.C, 186, 269
Chayovan, N, 159, 223
Chege, J.N, 322
Chimere-Dan, O, 323
Cho, L, 160
Choe, H.C, 172
Chojnacka, H, 324
Chowdhury, J, 142
Chuzhu, Z, 191
Clarke, J.I, 216
Cleland, J, 014, 161-163, 325, 456-457
Coale, A. J, 015, 164, 458
Cochraine, S.H, 016, 326
Cohen, B, 327
Concepcion, M.B, 165
Correa, C. S, 095
Courbage, Y, 166
Cross, A.R, 328
Curson, P, 216

Daily, G.C, 085
Das Gupta, M, 167-168
Dean, N.R, 329
Debavalya, N, 225
Degraff, D.S, 169
Demeny, P, 017, 459
Desta, Z, 330
Dharmalingam, A, 170
Diamond, I, 331-332
Diaz-Briquets, S, 064, 086
Dierckxsens, W, 065
Dimpa-Harry, S. H, 430
Dissanayake, L, 171
Dodoo, F.N, 333-337
Donaldson, L, 018
Donaldson, P.J, 172, 460
Douglas, R.M, 338
Dow, T.E, 339-341
Dowrick, S, 173
D'Souza, R.M, 338
Duraisamy, M, 174
Duryea, S, 094
Dwivedi, S.N, 175
Dyson, T, 019, 176-177
Dzekedzeke, K, 342

Easterlin, R, 020-021
Ebanks, G.E, 066-067
Economist, 343
Egero, B, 022, 168, 221, 344, 461
Ehrlich, P.R, 085
Eickelman, C, 178
Ekouevi, K, 345
El-Badry, M.A, 462
Emeruem, J.O, 430
Espenshade, T.J, 150

Fairlamb, C.D, 346
Farid, S.M, 326
Farooq, G.M, 347

Fawcett, J.T, 179
Feeney, G, 180-184
Ferrando, D, 068
Feyisetan, B.J, 389
Florez, C.E, 069, 084
Foote, K.A, 013, 040
Ford, N, 280
Fort, A.L, 070
Foster, A, 357, 443
Frank, O, 348
Freedman, R, 023, 185-186, 463
Frejka, T, 071
Fuller, G, 072

Gaisie, S.K, 349
Gans, P, 452
Gbortsu, E, 407
George, P.M, 066-067
Gertler, P, 187
Goldani, A.M, 073
Goldberg, H.I, 350
Goldman, N, 491
Goldscheider, C, 188, 194
Goldscheider, F, 024
Goldstein, A, 189
Goldstein, M.C, 256
Gomez, V, 074
Gonzales-Cortez, G, 075
Gonzalez, G, 133
Gosal, G.S, 190
Gould, W.T.S, 351
Graham, D.H, 099
Greenhalgh, S, 025-027, 191, 192
Greenspan, A, 193
Guest, P, 194, 195, 199-202
Guilkey, D, 169, 352
Guirre, A, 107
Gule, G, 353
Guo, S, 137, 196
Gupta, M.D, 197-198
Gupta, Y.P, 264
Guzman, J, 076-078, 113, 116, 136

Haghshenas, H, 079
Hailemariam, A, 354
Hammarskjold, M, 168, 221, 344, 461
Hammerslough, C.R, 355
Handwerker, W.P, 080-082
Harbison, S.F, 356, 424
Hashemi, S.M, 262
Havanon, N, 222, 224
Hayase, Y, 377, 470
Henriques, M.H, 122
Henry, L, 028
Hermalin, A.I, 046
Hertrich, V, 296, 383
Hicks, W.W, 083
Hilderink, H.B.M, 205
Hill, K, 107, 464
Hill, K.H, 357
Hill, R, 142
Hinde, P.R.A, 394-395
Hirschman, C, 199-202
Hobcraft, J, 456
Hogan, D, 084
Holl, K.D, 085
Hollerbach, P.E, 086
Horiuchi, S, 465
Hosaain, S.I, 203
Hull, T.H, 204
Hunter, I, 205
Hutaserani, S, 206

Institute of Resource Development (IRD) Macro International, 207, 358
Inter-American Development Bank, 087
Irfan, M, 263
Isiugo-Abanihe, U.C, 359
Iverson, S.B, 466

Jain, A.K, 208, 209
James, K.S, 210

James, W.H, 088
Jayatilake, M.J.J, 211
Jayne, S, 352
Jeffrey, R, 212
Jejeebhoy, S.J, 213
Jensen, A.M, 360-367
Jianhua, Y, 183
Jolly, C, 305, 379
Jones, G.W, 214-215, 338
Jones, H, 369
Jones, W.R, 089
Journal of International Development, 368
Jowett, A.J, 216
Juarez, F, 090

Kabir, M, 142
Kak, N, 245
Kalipeni, E, 370-372
Kalule, J.K, 375
Kamal, G.M, 162
Kamuansilpa, P, 159
Kamuzora, C.L, 378
Kaplan, H, 029
Karmal, G.M, 163
Karra, M.V, 217
Kates, R.W, 030
Kaufman, G, 091-092
Kayastha, S.L, 216
Kekovole, J, 340-341
Kelley, A.C, 373
Kertzer, D.I, 031
Keyfitz, N, 467
Khan, M.A, 226
Khander, S.R, 218
Khasakhala, A.A, 367
Khasiani, S, 340
Khoo, S.E, 179
Kibet, M, 376
Kidane, A, 374
Kim, D, 219
Kim, I, 220
Kirk, D, 032, 106
Kisanje, M, 375
Kishor, S, 221
Kizito, P, 328, 376
Klijzing, F, 093
Knodel, J, 159, 222-225, 246, 251
Kobayashi, K, 160
Kocher, J.E, 468
Koening, M.A, 226, 252
Kojima, H, 377
Komba, A, 378
Kono, S, 377, 469-471
Kreager, P, 033
Kumaran, T.V, 227

Ladier-Fouladi, M, 228
Lam, D.G.S, 094
Landers, J, 034
Latif, M.A, 218
Lavely, W.R, 229
Lee, B. S, 472
Lee, R.D, 013, 040
Lee-Jay, C, 233
Leete, R, 230-232
Le Grand, T.K, 234
Lesthaeghe, R.J, 035, 298, 379
Letamo, G, 380
Le Vine, R.A, 095
Le Vine, S.E, 095
Lewis, S, 254
Li, N, 191-192
Li, W, 235
Li, W.L, 236
Liang, Z, 235
Limanonda, B, 237
Lipton, M, 275
Llera, S, 090
Lockhood, M, 381
Locoh, T, 296, 382-383
Louis, G.P, 472
Loyola, M.A, 096
Loyola, R.B, 384
Lucas, D, 385-386
Lund, R, 238

Lutz, W, 165

Macro International, DHS, 387
Mahadevan, K, 239
Makinwa-Adebusoye, P, 388-389
Malmberg, B, 036
Manatou, J.M, 097
Mari Bhat, P.N, 198
Martin, C.T, 403
Martin, L.G, 233
Martine, G, 098
Mason, A, 157, 473
Mason, K.O, 037-039, 259
Maudin, W.P, 474, 485-486
Mazur, R.E, 390
Mbacke, C, 391
Mbizvo, M, 283-285
Mburugu, E, 344
McHenry, J.P, 475
McNeil, M, 350
McNicoll, G, 240-241, 476
Merrick, T, 099-101
Mhloyi, M.M, 390, 392-393
Mita, R, 242
Moini, R, 249
Molyneaux, J, 187
Montgomery, M.R, 040, 243, 298
Moore, M, 176
Moreno, L, 102-103, 137, 491
Morgan, S.P, 170, 244, 247
Morris, L, 483
Mturi, A.J, 394, 395
Muganzi, Z, 396
Muhuri, P.K, 477
Muhwava, W.B, 397
Mukiza-Gapere, J, 357
Muller, P.M, 095
Mundigo, A, 104
Murphy, M, 019, 177
Muvandi, I, 397, 437

Nabila, J.S, 300
Nag, M, 245
Nag, P, 216
National Council for Population and Development (NCPD) Kenya, 398-399
Nelson, N, 342
New York Times International, 400
Ngom, P, 401
Nguyen, V.P, 246
Nicholas, D.J, 172
Niessen, L.W, 205
Nieuwoudt, W.L, 346
Niraula, B.B, 244, 247
Njogu, W, 376, 402-403
Nkrumah, M, 404
Nobbe, C.E, 066-067, 373
Noble, J, 105
Norbert, S.A, 227
Notestein, F, 041

Obungu, W, 328, 376
Odaman, O.M, 405
Oechsli, F.W, 106
Oeppen, J, 054
Ofosu, Y, 478
Ogino, M, 248
Oheneba-Sakyi, Y, 406-407, 432
Omideyi, A.K, 408
Omondi-Odhiambo, 409
Omran, A.R, 042
Onuoha, N, 325, 410-411
Oppong, C, 390
Ordonez, G.M, 112
Orubuloye, I, 316, 318, 412
Osei-Hwedie, B, 413
Osei-Hwedie, K, 413
Osman, E.A, 414

Paiva, P.D.A, 060
Palloni, A, 107
Pantelides, E, 063, 078, 108, 113, 116, 136
Pardoe, M, 054
Parr, N.J, 415
Parrado, E.A, 109

Paxson, C.H, 357
Paydarfar, A.A, 249
Perez, L, 064
Pernia, E.M, 157
Peterson, K.D, 250
Phai, N.V, 251
Phillips, D, 479
Phillips, J.F, 162-163, 226, 234, 252
Pillet, B.D, 110
Pinto, G, 107
Pollak, R, 021, 043
Pong, S, 253
Population Division of the Department of International Economic and Social Affairs, UN Secretariat, 480
Population Impact Project (PIP) University of Ghana, 416
Population Reference Bureau, 111, 417-418
Potter, J.E, 044, 055, 112
Potts, M, 105
Poukouta, P, 419
Prada-Salas, E, 113
Pramualratana, A, 224
Price, N, 273, 420
Pullum, T.W, 263

Raftery, A.E, 254
Rai, S, 175
Ratcliffe, J, 255
Reddy, P.H, 155
Renne, E.P, 421-422
Repetto, R, 481
Retherford, R, 045
Richman, A, 095
Riley, A.P, 046, 262
Riley, N.E, 482
Rios, R, 114
Robey, B, 483-484
Robinson, W.C, 047, 356, 423-424
Rodriguez, G, 063, 078, 113, 115-116, 136, 295, 446
Rodriguez, J, 076
Rosero-Bixby, L, 046, 048, 117-120
Ross, J.A, 474, 485-486
Ross, J.L, 256
Roumasset, J, 206
Rustein, S.O, 302, 477, 483
Rutenberg, N, 331-332, 425

Safilios-Rothschild, C, 426
Salaff, J.W, 257
Sathar, Z.A, 258-259
Savitri, R, 260
Saw, S.H, 261
Sawyer, D.R, 060
Schkolnik, S, 063
Schuler, S, 256, 262
Schultz, T.P, 041, 299
Scriber, S, 427
Sedgh, G, 123
Seiver, D.A, 121
Shah, I.H, 263
Shapiro, D, 428-429, 433
Sharma, B.B.L, 264
Sharma, S, 264
Silva, N.V, 122
Simmons, R.S, 226, 242, 252, 265
Singh, R, 487
Singh, S, 063, 078, 102, 113, 116, 123
Singhal, D.S, 264
Siriboon, S, 223
Sittitrai, W, 222
Smith, H.L, 049
Sokari-George, E, 430
Song, R, 267
Songsore, J. S, 300
Soon, L, 266
Souza, A, 122
Spitz, A, 350
Stark, N.N, 217
Statistical Service of Ghana, 431
Stephen, L. S, 124

Stokes, C, 050
Studies in Family Planning, 125
Stycos, J.M, 126-127
Sudan, F.K, 268
Sumangala, M, 239
Sun, T.H, 187, 269
Surbakti, S, 270
Surkyn, J, 035
Szreter, S, 051

Takyi, B.A, 432
Tambashe, B.O, 428, 433
Tan, J, 201-202
Tanzania Bureau of Statistics, 434
Tapia, U.F.M, 095
Tawiah, E.O, 435
Taylor, A, 128
Taylor, H, 093
Teitelbaum, M, 488
Thangkasemvathana, B, 271
Thomas, D, 436-437
Thomas, N, 272-273
Tienda, M, 109
Timaeus, I.N, 325, 411
Timothy, T, 396
Torrez, P.H, 129
Tsui, A.O, 460
Tung, S.L, 130

Uddin, M.M, 274
Udjo, E.O, 438-439
Uitto, J, 489
Uitto, J.I, 440
United Nations, 132
United Nations Department for Economic and Social Information and Policy Analysis, 131
United Nations Economic Commission for Africa (ECA), 441
Uthoff, A, 133

Van Cam, M, 246, 251
Van de Kaa, D, 052
Vanderpost, C, 442
Van de Walle, E, 053, 443
Van Rompaey, S.E, 134
Verdugo, L.A, 135
Vosti, S.A, 275

Wang, F, 180, 189, 276
Ware, H, 444
Watcher, M.L, 021
Watkins, S, 005, 043, 490
Wawer, M.J, 298
Weinberger, M.B, 136
Werner, L.H, 339
Westley, S.B, 277
Westoff, C, 295, 445-446, 491
White, M.J, 137
Willekens, F.J, 205
Wilson, C, 014, 054
Wirakartakusmah, M.D, 278
Wolf, J, 217
Wong, L.R, 061
Wortham, R, 448-449

Xiao, B, 180
Xuyen, H, 246, 251

Yamuah, M, 450
Yang, M, 308
Yang, S, 279
Yankson, P.W.K, 300
Yasuko, H, 469
Yuma, M.N, 360

Zafar, M, 280
Zavala de Cosio, 138
Zhou, L, 281
Zhou, M, 180
Zhu, C, 192
Zhu, F, 282
Zhu, H, 279
Zlotnik, H, 139

Subject Index

(Based on Entry Numbers in the Text)

Acquired immune deficiency syndrome (AIDS), 150, 309
Abortifacient, 291
Abortion, 123, 160, 172, 283; induced, 004, 070
Adolescence, 020-021; and childbearing, 113
Age at first birth, 445
Agency and fertility, 011
Agricultural technology, 275
Antigua, 081, 082
Argentina, 108
Attitudinal change, 284
Autonomy of women. *See* Female autonomy

Bali, 231
Bangladesh: agrarian change, 153; contraception, 142, 218; contraceptive services, 252; contraceptive use, 226, 262; credit programmes, 262; culture, 272; diffusion, 242; economic security, 161, 272; education, 142; family planning programme, 163, 234, 274; family size preferences, 226; infant and child mortality, 234; poverty, 274; proximate determinants, 162; public programmes, 203; qualitative analysis of fertility, 265; risk and insurance, 153; socio-economic development, 274; women's role and status, 262
Barbados, 067, 080-081, 089, 124, 466
Birth control, 012, 062, 076, 098, 117, 163, 170, 344, 460; methods, 153. *See also* Contraception; Contraceptive (s)
Bolivia, 088, 129
Botswana: contraceptive use, 427; diffusion, 442; drought, 332, 419; economic crisis, 331; education, 436; family size, 321; fertility estimates, 311; proximate determinants, 380; sex preference, 321; westernization, 442
Brazil: abortion,123; contraception, 056; contraceptive methods, 092; contraceptive use, 123; culture, 122; development policies, 075; economic boom, 060; economic crisis, 061, 098; economic development, 099; education, 122, 135; family planning, 092; family planning programs, 487;

government policy, 062; ideational change, 122; infant mortality, 096; mass media, 098; mortality trends, 099; place of residence, 135; political economy, 059; proletarianization, 079; public policy, 057; religion, 122; Sao Paulo, 135; social inequality, 060; social institutions, 096; social organisation, 059; women's life course transitions, 073
Breast-feeding, 070, 376; prevalence, 258
British Carribean, 066
Burkina Faso, 447
Burundi, 427

Cameroon, 472
Changing Resource Management practices, 238
Chicago Columbia model of fertility decline, 002; chicago school, 047
Childbearing adolescent, 113
Child rearing costs, 037, 258, 388
Children: value of, 077, 362, 420
Chile, 072, 075, 076, 134
China: birth planning, 192; child mortality, 276; controlled and uncontrolled fertility, 229; ethnic groups, 279; family planning policy, 282; family planning projects, 164; famine, 216; famine amenorrhoea, 216; mortality decline, 276; one child policy, 277; political economy, 192; population policy, 273; rural and urban China, 235; socio-economic development, 281; spousal separation, 216
Cohort shifts, 406
Colombia, 069, 076, 084, 090, 112, 113, 116, 138, 475, 487
Community development, 270
Consensual union, 109
Contraception, 160, 375, 415, 172, 221
Contraception, in: Asia, 158; Bangladesh, 162; East Asia, 160; Ghana, 415, 292, 336, 358, 425, 435; India, 221, 155; Kenya, 350; Korea, 172; Latin America, 136, 056, 071, 123; Nepal, 148. *See also* Birth control
Contraceptive (s): methods in : Asia, 158; Brazil, family planning and, 092; Ghana, 358; Latin America, 136; Zimbabwe, 283; use, 004, 065; use in: Africa, 298; Asia Pacific, 185; Bangladesh, 226; Kenya, 350, 355, 402; Nepal, 256; Peru, 070; Phillipines, 169; Southeast Asia, 165; Sub-Saharan Africa, 427; Taiwan, family planning, 186; Zimbabwe, 283. *See also* Contraception
Costa Rica: birth control, 076; catholic church, 085; diffusion, 117-118, 120, family planning, 127; family planning program, 065; literacy, 127; marriage patterns, 126; modernisation, 127; socio-economic development, 475; spatial dimensions, 093; status of women, 085; structural changes, 076; women's participation in economic activities, 133
Cote d' I voire, 290, 299, 427
Credit programmes, 218, 262
Cuba, 064, 075, 086, 105
Culture, 026, 030, 038, 372; change, 239; factors, 145, 176; forces, 009; norms, 018; setting, 286

Demand theory, 215
Demographic transition, 030, 033, 034, 042, 093, 140, 173; theory, 023, 042, 050, 051, 058
Development: planning, 144;

policies, 075, 381; economic, 083, 187
Diffusion: 038, 058, 065; adaptation, 012; of birth control, 045; effects, 048; family planning information, 242; innovation, 012; of new ideas, 242; social, 115; study, 005; theory, 215
Domestic violence, 304
Dominican Republic, 090, 116
Drought, 331, 419

Early marriage. *See* Marriage
East Java, 231
Economic boom, 060
Economic crisis, 006, 098, 331, 332, 357, 473; international, 061
Economic development, 083
Economic and social development, 045, 143
Ecuador, 088, 090, 116
Education; 081, 082, 094, 210, 428; female school attendance and, 095; fertility and, 016; husband and, 284, 285; mass and, 008; women and, 037, 082, 109, 259, 299
Emigration and fertility decline, 067
Employment opportunities, 082, 428
Environmental impact assessment, 459
Environmental pressure, 371
Epidemiological transition model, 042
Ethiopia, 330, 354
Ethnic fertility differentials, 261
Ethnic groups, 279
External debt, 087

Family: background, 433; change, 312-313; economy, 257; emotional nucleation of the, 009, 339, 341; formation process, 090; household, 024, 037; income distribution, 069; life, 432; limitation, 053; organisation, 414; size, 114, 203, 222, 224, 312, 320, 423; size intentions, 257; structure, 156; welfare, 264
Family planning: efforts, 030; men's participation in, 217, 409; men's unmet need for, 401; methods, 264, 328; policy, 092, 258, 282; practices, 139; programs, 056, 065, 089, 104, 123, 154-155, 163, 165, 1765 187, 196, 218, 221, 226, 230, 234, 236, 245, 265, 269, 274, 281, 318, 319, 377, 391, 454-455; promotion, 293; provisions, 379; services, 085, 424; timing and spacing of births, 403
Famine, 216
Female autonomy: 176, 407; birth control and, 170; decision making and, 407; fertility and, 037, 190, 212, 244
Fertility decision making, 217
Focus group sessions and fertility transitions, 224, 265

Gambia, 450
Gender, 238, 322, 361, 390; relations, 322
Ghana: abortifacient, 291; child mortality, 415; communication programmes, 416; contraception, 291, 336, 358, 425, 435; contraceptive prevalence, 425; contraceptive use, 435; cultural setting, 286; decision making, 407; family life, 432; family planning programmes, 333; female autonomy, 407; fertility norm, 336; gender roles, 407; Greater Accra region, 415; income, 300; local herbs, 291; marriage, 432; place of residence, 415; proximate determinants, 415; religion, 415; reproductive cessation, 334; teenage fertility, 289; unmet need for men and women's contraceptive

behaviour, 337; women's education, 299
Guam, 130

Haiti, 125
Health transition, 042, 044
Herbs and fertility decline, 291
Honduras, 076
Hong Kong, 144, 160, 231, 479
Husband's education. *See* Education

Ideational change; and fertility, 035, 038, 122, 254; factors, 014; theory, 033
Illiteracy, 312
India: child mortality, 213; contraception, 155; culture, 145; development, 209; diffusion, 153; economic pressure, 241; education, 210; family planning, 277; family planning program, 209; family welfare, 264; female autonomy, 176; female literacy, 264; gender relations, 177; income, 264; infant mortality, 264; Kerela, 205; kinship structure, 176; marriage,145;mortality, 139; population growth, 139; population policy, 209; poverty, 264; risk and insurance, 153; social justice, 255; Tamil Nadu, 221; Uttar Pradesh, 205; women's autonomy, 212; women's choice of work, 170, 174
Indonesia, 187-188, 200, 204, 207, 240, 241, 270, 278, 469, 487
Industrialisation, 041
Infant and child mortality, 096, 138, 166, 209, 218, 234, 260, 296, 316
Informal sector, 065
Institutional approaches of fertility, 027, 215
Insurance against risk, 007
Intergenerational transfer of resources, 404
International migration. *See* Migration
Iran, 141, 228, 249, 254

Japan, 160, 182, 248, 469

Kenya: AIDS prevalence, 399; child mortality, 306, 363; contraceptive prevalence, 350; contraceptive use, 402; domestic violence, 304; empowerment of women, 304; family planning, 356; gender relations, 322; marriage, 324; nutrition, 360; population dynamics, 305; population policy, 351; proximate determinants of fertility, 376; racial patterns of fertility, 323; social value of children, 365; wealth flows, 303, 340-341
Kerela, 210, 239
Kinship structure, 176
Korea, 105, 144, 160, 172, 182, 188, 193, 219, 220, 231, 272, 472, 481

Labour force participation, 109, 173; of women, 109
Land tenure, 421
Life expectancy, 083, 140
Literacy, 126, 260

Madagascar, 447
Madhya Pradesh, 175
Malawi, 371, 372
Malaysia, 160, 200, 215, 232, 253, 261, 266
Mali, 308, 427
Marriage, 070, 432; early, 451; later age at, 138, 160, 166; patterns, 119, 230, 237; relations, 361
Mass media, 098, 293, 295, 377, 446, 447

Mauritius, 369, 466, 479
Mexico, 055, 083, 095, 097, 103, 110, 116, 121, 131, 472, 487
Micro economic data, 149
Micro economic theory of fertility, 047
Migration, 099, 137, 219, 307-308; internal, 214; international, 450; rural urban, 308
Modernisation, 106, 122, 127, 392, 442; process, 249
Mortality, 219, 220, 473; child, 299, 306, 367; decline, 045, 083, 101, 114, 207, 239, 277, 314; trends, 464

Namibia, 447
Natural fertility, 003, 028, 054, 213
Nepal, 146-149, 247, 256
New Home Economic model of fertility, 001
Nigeria: contraception, 347, 405, 428; Ekpoma region, 405; family limitation, 317; family planning program, 347; family planning promotion, 293; fertility desires, 294, 361; Ibadan city, 314, 317; land tenure, 421; marriage, 405, 422; mass media, 293, 295; nuclear family, 408; postpartum abstinence, 315; rural electrification, 430; Southwestern Nigeria, 316; sterility, 438
Nuclear family, 408
Nuptiality patterns. *See* Marriage patterns
Nutrition, 360; deprivation, 216

Oman, 178

Pakistan, 258-259, 263, 275, 280
Parity progression ratios, 181
Pennsylvania model of fertility, 021
Peru, 056, 068, 070, 088, 090, 116, 137
Phillipines, 169, 200, 204
Political economy of fertility, 025-027, 031, 059
Population: agency, 220, growth, 448 450, 465; policy, 056, 164-165, 195, 209, 274, 413; projections, 204
Postpartum: amenorrhoea, 283; infecundability, 004, 376, 378
Poverty, 264; urban, 099
Proletarianization process, 079
Proximate determinants of fertility, 004, 086, 102, 162, 246, 380, 410, 415
Public programmes, 203
Puerto Rico, 481
Punjab, 168, 221, 245, 344, 461

Qualitative analysis of fertility transition, 224
Quantum and tempo of fertility, 389

Racial patterns of fertility decline, 324
Regional fertility patterns, 442
Relative income hypothesis of fertility, 020
Replacement level fertility, 052, 082, 140, 159, 182-183, 288
Reproductive decision making, 359
Role of women, 362
Rural development programme, 147, 394, 414
Rural electrification, 430
Rural income generating programs, 147
Rwanda, 382

Senegal, 308, 410-411, 427
Sex bias, 198
Sex preference, 247, 253, 320,
Sexual abstinence, 315
Sierra Leone, 321
Singapore, 144, 160, 179, 193, 204, 215, 231, 257, 212
Social change, 079, 146, 178, 223,

372, 440
Social context, 194
Social development, 239
Social inequality, 060
Social influence, 040
Social interaction, 048, 117-118, 120
Social justice, 255
Social learning, 040
Social networks, 005
Socio-economic change, 356
Socio-economic development, 110, 112, 189
South Africa, 323, 353
Spatial analysis of fertility, 236, 288
Spousal separation, 308
Sri Lanka, 156, 171, 211, 231, 238, 250, 469, 475, 487
Structural adjustment policies, 345
Structural change of family economy, 014; Latin American society, 076
Structural determinants of fertility, 169
Sudan, 414
Survival: child, 042, 095, 335
Swaziland, 450

Taiwan: contraception, 469; diffusion, 243; economic security, 272; economic development, 144; education, 236; family planning program, 186, 236, 269; infant mortality, 236; marriage, 160
Tamil Nadu, 221, 227, 260, 344, 461
Tanzania, 378, 394, 395, 427, 434
Thailand: AIDS epidemic, 150; Bali, 231; culture, 160; East Java, 231; epidemiological transition, 479; family planning, 237; family planning program, 237; nuptiality change, 237
Timing and spacing of birth. *See also* Family planning
Togo, 308, 382, 427
Trinidad and Tobago, 116

Uganda, 308, 375, 427
Urban elite, 312, 313
Urbanisation, 041
Urban middle class, 284
Urban poverty, 099

Venezuela, 109
Vietnam, 204, 246, 251

War, 325
Wealth flows, 009, 029, 303, 340, 341; intergenerational, 404
Westernisation, 442
Women: autonomy, *See* Female autonomy; choice of work, 174; empowerment, 304; income, 426; labour force participation, 109; life course transitions, 073; participation in economic activities, 133; social value, 362; status of, 085, 131, 134, 166; work, 170, 394

Zaire, 428, 429, 433
Zambia, 342, 413, 447
Zimbabwe: contraception, 284, 352, 439; education, 285, 436; family planning, 352, 487; gender equality 284; population policies, 427; proximate determinants, 397; sampling, 437; socio-economic factors, 393; structural and attitudinal change, 283; women's work, 390

About the Compiler

SAMUEL AGYEI-MENSAH is a lecturer in the Department of Geography and Resource Development at the University of Ghana. He has published a number of articles on population and the geography of health.

CPSIA information can be obtained at www.ICGtesting.com
Printed in the USA
LVOW040821301112

309428LV00005B/27/P

9 780313 302428